W9-DAE-108

KEYS TO MENOPAUSE AND BEYOND

Elizabeth Vierck

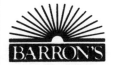

BARRON'S

UCC LIBRARY
ELIZABETH CAMPUS

To my sister and other women friends who are making this hormone passage with me.

I am indebted to Kip Wotkyns for his interest and contributions, particularly in the "Questions That Men Ask" section.

The passage in the Foreword is from *Fried Green Tomatoes at the Whistle Stop Cafe* by Fannie Flagg.
Copyright © 1987 by Fannie Flagg.
Reprinted by permission of Random House, Inc.

© Copyright 1992 by Barron's Educational Series, Inc.

All rights reserved.
No part of this book may be reproduced in any form, by photostat, microfilm, xerography, or any other means, or incorporated into any information retrieval system, electronic or mechanical, without the written permission of the copyright owner.

All inquiries should be addressed to:
Barron's Educational Series, Inc.
250 Wireless Boulevard
Hauppauge, New York 11788

Library of Congress Catalog Card No. 92-309

International Standard Book No. 0-8120-4994-2

Library of Congress Cataloging-in-Publication Data

Vierck, Elizabeth, 1945–
    Keys to menopause and beyond / Elizabeth Vierck.
        p.   cm.—(Barron's retirement keys)
    Includes bibliographical references (p.   ) and index.
    ISBN 0-8120-4994-2
    1. Menopause—Popular works.   I. Title. II. Series.
RG186.V54   1992
618.1'75—dc20
                                          92-309
                                          CIP

PRINTED IN THE UNITED STATES OF AMERICA
234   5500   987654321

618.1
Vi 676

CONTENTS

FOREWORD

"Oh, Mrs. Threadgoode, I'm too young to be old and too old to be young. I just don't fit anywhere. I wish I could kill myself, but I don't have the courage."

Mrs. Threadgoode was appalled. "Why, Evelyn Couch, you mustn't even think such a thing. That's like sticking a sword in the side of Jesus!! That's just silly talk, honey—you've just got to pull yourself together and open your heart to the Lord. He'll help you.

Now, let me ask you this. Are your breasts sore?"

Evelyn looked at her. "Well, sometimes."

"Does your back and legs ache?"

"Yes. How did you know?"

"Simple, honey. You're just going through a bad case of menapause, that's all that's the matter with you. What you need is to take your hormones and to get out every day and walk in the fresh air and walk yourself right through it. That's what I did when I was in it. I used to burst into tears eating a steak, just thinkin' about that poor cow. I like to have drove Cleo crazy, crying all the time, thinking nobody loved me....

"I got out and walked every day, alongside the railroad tracks, up and down, just like we're doing now, and pretty soon I had walked my way right through it and I was back to normal."

"But, I thought I was too young to be going through it," Evelyn said. "I just turned forty-eight."

"Oh no, honey, lots of women go through it early."...

"Do you really think that's what's the matter with me? Is that why I've been so irritable?"

"Sure it is. Oh, it's worse than a merry-go-round…up and down, down and up."

from *Fried Green Tomatoes at the Whistle Stop Cafe*
by Fannie Flagg. Copyright © 1987 by Fannie Flagg.
Reprinted by permission of Random House, Inc.

Like Evelyn, I had spent the summer going up and down, down and up. I thought that I was going crazy—every small annoyance was an occasion for clenched teeth, every encounter an opportunity for a snide comment. Life wore fangs and I was its victim. I told myself that my grudges and outbursts, my anxiety and depression were justified—a disorganized, noisy renovation was going on in my home and work environment; my mother fell and broke her hip after a spat with an incompetent caregiver; I had not totally recovered from a couple of miscarriages. However, none of these occurrences normally would have elicited the irritability and outbursts that had become my hallmark.

I did not know that I was experiencing the effects of oscillating hormones. At the time the thought that I might be entering menopause never occurred to me. I was 46 and had been told by a number of doctors that I could expect to begin the change in my mid-fifties, at about the age that my mother and sister went through it. I thought that I had another seven or eight years before I had to think about it, much less experience it.

When I first learned that I was in early menopause, I was stunned. Quickly, my reaction plummeted to depression and anger. My images of menopause were dark and gloomy. Out of my long list of fears and prejudices, my husband's favorite was my assumption that, after menopause, all women become short and round. (I have watched several women friends shrink into beach balls when they reached menopause age. Unhappily, there is some truth to this likeness and it is particularly important to pay attention to diet and exercise during and after these years.)

But my depression centered around my perception that, with my body's decrease in estrogen production, a number of doors were slamming shut. For example, my husband and I would have to give up all hope of having a child. (When I mention this concern to older women who had their babies in their twenties, they look at me as if I were crazy to even consider getting pregnant in my mid-forties. But I had always been a late bloomer. In fact, a number of my friends had been able to pull off pregnancies in their forties, and an obstetrician friend of mine had a patient who had her first child at 48. I assumed that I could be one of these exceptions.)

I also felt the cold wind blowing against the gateway to my youth. I felt age rage (and, I am a gerontologist!). I began to worry about what it would be like to work with men my age and ten, twenty, or thirty years younger. Would they judge my work as that of an old lady, rather than on its merits?

The cold wind also elicited what I will call life review—a hard look at what I've accomplished in relation to what I had expected to achieve. (I have since discovered that this sort of personal inventory is common during this period of life.)

Ultimately, the life review led to a wonderful, light feeling of renewal. With some adjustment to the estrogen therapy, my moods have calmed down significantly. According to statistics, I have about a third of my life ahead and I am looking forward to it with zest. I would like to share with you three important tips based on my experience during this time:

The Man in Your Life

During my adjustment to menopause I was blessed with a number of emotional bolsterers: a supportive husband; a sister and women friends who listened to me endlessly; and a supportive doctor. I highly recommend all three.

First, if there is a man in your life, it is important to explain to him what you are going through. (You may want to show him the "Questions That Men Ask" section on page 140 of this book, and then talk it over.) He should know that some very real changes are occurring in your body and that you are experiencing some very strange sensations. I remember one time, for instance, when my husband walked into the kitchen where I was standing, looking as if I had just crawled out of a full kitchen sink. I was soaked from head to toe. "It's not that hot in here," he said. "Low blood sugar," I said. (At the time that's all I could think of to explain this curious, hot shakiness that occasionally possessed my body.)

I also remember padding through the house at all hours of the night and early morning, because of a ghostly wakefulness that pulled me out of a comfortable sleep. Eventually, I didn't even expect to sleep through the night. Later, I could explain these alien reactions and behaviors to my husband in relation to my raging hormones, and there was relief on both our parts that it wasn't our relationship that was causing these anxiety-like states.

A word of warning: You can expect the man in your life to feel some embarrassment when the "m" word first comes up. For example, when I first started on my menopause journey, if my husband and I were in a restaurant or other public place and I uttered the "m" word, he would look around with embarrassment to see if anyone had overheard me. (In all fairness this reaction is not limited to men; Susan, one of my most enlightened female friends, does the same thing.) Now, he has gotten used to and accepted this ongoing chatter about hot flashes and estrogen levels.

Women Friends

I can't say enough about my sister and women friends who have listened to my fright and fears as I have gone through this passage. There is nothing like talking to another woman who can relate to the trauma of hot flashes, drying "privates," and sleepless nights. My advice is gather up these valued companions in this journey and talk their heads off. You'll feel better and they'll feel better because of the camaraderie. Talk to women your age who are going through menopause and to women who went through it a decade or more ago.

Doctors

I am very fortunate because I have a doctor I can relate to and with whom I can share my fears honestly. My doctor understands, is even fascinated by, what our raging hormones do to us during menopause. Her sympathetic attitude has made this passage far easier than it would be otherwise. But, unhappily, she is an exception. Too many doctors still think that the symptoms of menopause are "just midlife stress." I believe that if your physician doesn't give you enough time to listen to your symptoms, won't help you find the best possible hormone dosage that works for you, or suggests that any of your symptoms are "just in your mind," you should look for a new doctor.

How to Use This Book

When I told my doctor that I was writing this book, she made this very important point: "Tell them that menopause will affect them for the rest of their lives, it is not just one shot in time."

In this spirit, this book is designed to be referred to again and again, not only as you approach and go through the change, but through your postmenopause years, as the need arises. It includes important information for women on a range of topics such as how to perform breast self-exams, the types of cancers to watch out for, and how to add calcium and fiber to your diet.

It is my hope that the information here will dispel many of the myths about menopause and that you will take advantage of the many options for lessening the negative impact of menopause.

1

MENOPAUSE—THE EXPERIENCE

Some of us are miserable as we go through menopause; others never notice a thing. Some of us mourn the passing of the eggs; others love the freedom that comes with not worrying about getting pregnant. Some of us can't wait to get on estrogen; others are scared to death to take hormones.

Menopause is common to all women who are beyond their reproductive years. But the experience is unique for each of us. This Key describes the diversity of the menopause experience as told by women themselves, starting with that of women who are now in their sixties and then providing snapshots of women who are in their forties and fifties.

While I was writing this book, a friend of mine invited me to attend a meeting of her women's group, which had been getting together one Saturday a month for close to twenty years. Most of the women in the group were in their early sixties. They were all energetic, loving women. The group had gone through births, miscarriages, illnesses, deaths, divorces, firings, and hirings. They had had lengthy talks about women's issues. But they had never discussed menopause. In fact, it became very clear to me, after listening to these vital women, that menopause was a closed topic during their era and it was assumed that most symptoms were "just in the mind." And their doctors, all of whom were men, reinforced this assumption. Here are five of their stories.

Joan remembers with agony the three-day hiking trip she took with her husband and several other couples. On the first day, as she was ascending a mountain, blood started to pour out of her and soaked through her only pair of jeans. It did not stop gushing for two unbearable days. Another woman, Betty,

1

had a similar experience, but instead of blood, it was sweat that streamed over her body and down her legs.

Two other women, Esther and Jane, related that they had unbearable, blinding headaches at the time they were going through "the change." Both of their doctors said the headaches were "just stress." The word *menopause* was never mentioned. In fact, because they both had a lot of other things going on in their lives and no one told them that headaches sometimes went along with menopause, they had never associated the two—until now, when they look back with agony. Jane put it this way: "Wow, my menopause was very difficult. I was really very miserable during that period in my life."

Roberta, on the other hand, breezed through menopause over a decade ago without a hot flash, headache, or any other symptom. She had no idea what her friends were talking about when they groaned over their "night sweats," sighed over their waning libidos, or discussed any of the other symptoms of menopause. Roberta has never taken estrogen and, so far, has no sign of osteoporosis or heart disease.

The other women I talked to, who ranged in age from 35 to 55, have had the advantage of a slightly more open attitude toward menopause and an increasing understanding of the physiological basis for the symptoms that go along with it. However, their experiences reflect the same diversity as the older group. Here are some snapshots.

- Sonia, age 35, went into an instant menopause because of a hysterectomy and was out of work for a month because of severe hot flashes and headaches. Finally she found an estrogen dosage that worked for her, relieving most symptoms.
- Beth, age 48, had miserable symptoms for over a year and found tremendous relief from taking estrogen, only to seriously rebound when she added progesterone during the last days of the month. Finally, taking a lower, daily dosage of progesterone helped solve the problem, but she still does not feel back to normal.

- Laura, age 55, just stopped having periods. Her biggest problem is with facial hair and gaining weight, but she has never had a hot flash or a sleepless night.
- Tammy, age 56, has shrunk two inches in the last three years and cannot take hormones because of a family history of estrogen-dependent breast cancer. She is worried about osteoporosis.

Your experience with menopause may or may not be similar to that of one of these women. You may be one of the lucky 15 percent who have no symptoms, the 70 percent who experience some symptoms but are not too miserable, or the unlucky 15 percent who have severe symptoms. Whatever your overt symptoms, it is important to remember that the changes taking place in your body are as significant as those you went through in puberty. Fortunately, there are many things that can be done to adjust to them, the majority of which are described in this book. In fact, your approach to reading this book might be to first read over those Keys that apply to your specific symptoms. But be sure also to look carefully at the sections that focus on the long-term effects of estrogen depletion, such as Key 18 on osteoporosis and Key 37 on women and heart disease.

Ultimately, when the adjustment to menopause is made well, the result is midlife vitality. No one has said it better than Margaret Mead: "The most creative force in the world is the menopausal woman with zest."

AVERAGE AGE OF ONSET OF
ESTROGEN-DEFICIENCY PROBLEMS

Problem	Age
MENSTRUAL CHANGES	~49
HOT FLASHES	~51
VAGINAL THINNING	~52
BLADDER PROBLEMS	~53
SKIN CHANGES	~54
LOSS OF URINE	~55
OSTEOPOROSIS	~59
CIRCULATION PROBLEMS	~64

Age: 45 50 55 60 65 70

Source: *Medfax-Sentinel*

4

2

WHAT IS MENOPAUSE?

What is menopause? To you it may mean hot flashes, sleep disturbances, and depression, while your closest friend breezes through it without noticing anything but a decrease in her periods. Because menopause is a period in your life when specific changes are taking place in your body, and there is tremendous variability in the way individuals respond to these changes, it is important to understand what menopause is and how to recognize it.

Many women experience the hot flashes, headaches, mood swings, and other symptoms of menopause and, not realizing what is happening to them, feel stressed by the strange changes that are occurring in their bodies. "I thought I was going crazy," relates one 42-year-old woman who went into an early menopause. "I would wake up at night with a blinding headache, drenched in sweat. The next day I would think it was all in my mind." Once she understood what was causing her problem and how to treat it, her stress was greatly relieved.

What specifically causes the problem? Decreasing levels of the hormone estrogen. Estrogen is a powerful hormone, and its depletion causes long-lasting, dramatic changes to the body's skin, muscles, tissues, and bones. These changes may be noticed a few months after the last period. Specifically, here are some of the major changes that occur for all women during menopause:[1]

• The ovaries shrink and stop producing eggs, resulting in infertility and cessation of menstrual periods.

---

[1]Based in part on Morton A. Stenchever and George Aagaard, *Caring for the Older Woman* (New York: Elsevier, 1991), p. 207.

- The vagina becomes dry and the walls of the vagina thin out and lose elasticity.
- The lining of the uterus, the endometrium, thins and shrinks.
- The urethra shrinks and its tissues thin out.
- The breasts lose their layer of subcutaneous fat and glandular tissue shrinks, causing them to droop.
- The skin loses moisture and its subcutaneous fat.
- Muscles lose tone.
- Bone mass decreases, greatly increasing the risk for osteoporosis.
- The tissue supports for many organs such as the vagina and bladder become weak, causing them to relax.
- LDL, the "bad cholesterol," increases.
- Vascular changes occur, causing hot flashes.

The good news is that, for women who can take hormone replacement therapy, most of these changes can be held off or reversed.

Symptoms of Menopause

Due to the loss of estrogen, certain physical signs or symptoms of menopause occur. Some lucky women never have real problems with these changes, because their ovaries, adrenal glands, and fat tissue continue to produce enough estrogen after menopause that the symptoms occur more slowly and easily. However, most women will experience at least three or four of the major signs of menopause listed below. Details of these symptoms are described in Keys 9 through 17.

- Hot flashes or flushes
- Changes in menstruation
- Vaginal changes
- Stress incontinence
- Weight gain
- Skin and hair changes
- Premenstrual syndrome
- Sleep changes

- Mood swings
- Osteoporosis

Other Physical Changes

Other symptoms can also occur leading up to and during menopause, although they are less common. Women sometimes complain of migraine headaches, dizziness, and heart palpitations. Other signs include aching joints, cold hands and feet (regardless of the weather), fatigue, lethargy, jitters, shortness of breath, and a feeling as if insects are crawling all over them.

The Demographics of Menopause

According to Dr. Wulf H. Utian of the University Hospitals in Cleveland, a pioneer on research on menopause, in the next ten years there are going to be more women going through menopause than at any other time in history. In the next ten years, 50 million women will go through menopause.[2] Based on average statistics, half of all women will stop menstruating by age 48, and by age 52, 85 percent will have reached menopause.[3]

Overcoming Fears:

As described in the foreword, many women feel uneasy about menopause. However, although some inevitable changes do take place during the climacteric, the effects of most can be alleviated with proper treatment and preventive care. The following Keys will focus on preparing for these changes and making the most of the menopausal and postmenopausal years.

---

[2]Dr. Wulf H. Utian, quoted in Jerry E. Bishop, "Doubt Remains About Estrogen for Menopause," *Wall Street Journal*, September 12, 1991, p. B1.

[3]University of California at Berkeley, *The Wellness Encyclopedia* (Boston: Houghton Mifflin, 1991) p. 365.

3

THE STAGES OF MENOPAUSE

The Climacteric

A number of terms are used to describe the years surrounding menopause. For example, if you are under age 40 and you are in menopause, your doctor may refer to your condition as a premature menopause. (Premature menopause is described in Key 7.) If you are in your forties, your doctor may tell you that you are perimenopausal, premenopausal, or beginning the climacteric. Then, when you reach your fifties, the description will change to menopausal or postmenopausal.

All of these terms describe part of a decade-plus process called the climacteric or change of life. They describe the fact that changes in the female reproductive system are going on throughout midlife. The climacteric, or climacterium refers to the span of years over which a woman's reproductive stage ends. These years often begin at age 35 to 40 and end at ages 50 to 55. During the climacteric, specific changes take place—most notably, hormone levels drop, the ovaries gradually stop producing eggs, periods become irregular, and eventually they stop entirely.

Although it is popular to describe this entire period as menopause, it is just one of four stages of the climacteric, which includes premenopause, perimenopause, menopause, and postmenopause. Each stage has its own characteristic changes.

Premenopause is the first stage of the climacteric, when symptoms often begin to appear, such as irregular periods. This period may span months, years, or even a decade.

Perimenopause is the period preceding the time when periods stop entirely. During the perimenopause many months may go by between periods before they stop.

8

Menopause is the term used to describe that specific point in time when you had your last period.

Postmenopause occurs when you have not had a period in at least a year.

How Your Doctor Determines If You Are in Menopause

To the physician, menopause is the time when your ability to reproduce ends. In medical terms, your official date of menopause is the date of your final menstrual period. The usual age of occurrence is between 48 and 55 years. The median age is 51.4 years.

The first sign of menopause that usually occurs is a change in the frequency and flow of menstrual periods. If you are in your forties or fifties and you notice a change in the frequency and flow of your periods, or any of the other common symptoms described above, your doctor should perform some specific tests to officially diagnose your condition.

To determine whether you are approaching or in menopause, your doctor may take samples of your blood to look at levels of two pituitary hormones that are elevated during menopause. The hormones are called LH (luteinizing hormone) and FSH (follicle-stimulating hormone). Your doctor may also take some cells from your vagina to estimate your hormone levels. This is called vaginal cytology.

4

THE MYTHS VS. THE
REALITY OF MENOPAUSE

Many of the fears that you undoubtedly have about menopause are based on myth. Will you lose your mind? Become sexless? Let's compare some feelings such as these with the realities of menopause.

Menopause is a disease. Menopause is not a disease. It is a stage in development that occurs for every woman. In fact, many health professionals do not like to refer to the "symptoms" of menopause because they feel that the word *symptoms* suggests that menopause is part of a disease process rather than a natural process. They prefer using the word *signs* to describe the hot flashes and related physical events caused by the reduction in hormone levels that occurs in menopause.

I'll become a crazy old lady. Women in menopause do not lose their minds, although many women in midlife do become more independent, more sure of themselves, and more in tune with their bodies. And for those women who do have mood swings caused by oscillating hormones, taking estrogen will greatly alleviate symptoms.

I'll no longer find sex exciting or desirable. With proper treatment, there is no reason for sex to become less enjoyable with menopause. In fact, many women report increased pleasure in sex during this time because of lack of fear of pregnancy.

I'm sure to have all those unpleasant symptoms. Fifteen percent of women have no symptoms, and only about another 15 percent experience severe symptoms. Eighty-five percent of women with symptoms can be helped with hormone replacement therapy.[1]

The symptoms of menopause are all in my head. While some symptoms may be related to emotions, none are imaginary. However, natural, dramatic processes are going on in the body and with them come physical reactions like hot flashes, palpitations of the heart, and thinning of the skin.

Menopause is the beginning of the decline into old age. Most women will have at least one-third, probably half, of their lives left after menopause. For many, these will be healthy and fulfilling years.

The body stops producing estrogen at menopause. The truth is that our estrogen production has been slowly decreasing since our mid-twenties, when production peaked and it was easiest to get pregnant. The body never entirely stops producing estrogen, but it does slow down.

If I take estrogen I'll get cancer. Many doctors feel that estrogen helps protect against cancer of the ovary, a more serious disease than uterine cancer.[2] With the addition of progesterone, the risk of developing uterine cancer has been greatly reduced. In fact, women who take estrogen have lower death rates from all causes than those who do not.

[1]Mary Beard and Lindsay Curtis, *Menopause and the Years Ahead* (Tucson: Fisher, 1988), p. 5.

[2]Niels Laursen and Steven Whitney, *A Woman's Body: The New Guide to Gynecology* (New York: Perigee, 1987), p. 431.

5

ABOUT THE REPRODUCTIVE SYSTEM

In order to appreciate what happens to the body during menopause, it is helpful to understand the reproductive cycle. Women come into the world with all of the potential for reproduction already formed, including about 5 million potential eggs, called *oocytes*. Our reproductive system matures as we mature. Men, on the other hand, produce new sperm throughout their lives.

The reproductive system is regulated by *hormones*, which are carried through the body in the blood and lymph system. The hormones that are important to our discussion of menopause are estrogen, testosterone, and progesterone. Most of the estrogen and progesterone is produced in the ovaries, which also produce some testosterone. Testosterone is important to women, as well as men.

Hormone levels begin to decline long before the symptoms of menopause occur. However, if the ovaries are surgically removed, estrogen levels will plummet. (For more information on hormones, see Key 6.)

External Genitourinary Organs

In women this area is known as the genitals, pubic area, or vulva. The organs are greatly affected by the loss of estrogen during menopause and consist of the following:
- The area of fatty tissue over the pubic bone, called the *mons veneris*, *mons pubis*, or *Mount of Venus*.
- The outer and inner lips, called the *labia majora* and *labia minora*. They protect the reproductive and urinary openings.
- The *clitoris*, a small, bud-shaped organ at the area where the inner lips join below the mons.

- The *vagina opening*, the entrance to the vagina.
- The *urethra*, the opening to the urinary passage and bladder.
- The *anus*, which leads to the rectum.

Internal Reproductive Organs

These organs are also greatly affected by estrogen depletion and menopause (see Fig. 1):

Figure 1

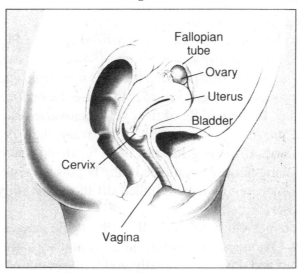

- The *vagina*, the canal lying between the rectum and the bladder. It is the area of the body where sexual intercourse occurs. It stretches easily during sex or childbirth.
- The *cervix*, the mouth of the uterus.
- The *uterus*, a pear-shaped organ about the size of a lemon. It carries the fetus during pregnancy.
- The *endometrium*, the mucous membrane lining of the uterus. It goes through changes as part of the menstrual cycle.

American College of Obstetricians and Gynecologists. *The Menopause Years.* AGOC Patient Education Pamphlet #47. Washington, DC © 1984.

13

- *Ovaries*, two small organs located on either side of the uterus. They produce eggs and the female sex hormones, estrogen and progesterone. During the reproductive years they release an ovum every month.
- The *fallopian tubes*, one on each side of the uterus. Eggs travel through the fallopian tubes from the ovary to the uterus.

The Menstrual Cycle

During the reproductive years, the endometrium builds up each month in order to receive a fertilized egg (see Fig. 2). If an egg is not fertilized, the lining is shed as a menstrual period. During the first part of a month's menstrual cycle, the ovaries produce estrogen in order to cause the endometrium to build up. In the middle of the cycle the ovaries release an egg and pregnancy may result. The ovary then produces progesterone. If the egg has not been fertilized, the ovaries stop releasing hormones and the lining begins to break down. The endometrium is then sloughed off in the monthly menstrual flow.

As you get close to your 40s, this cycle may become irregular. Ovulation may not occur at all and hormone levels may go up and down. Eventually you will run out of eggs.

Figure 2

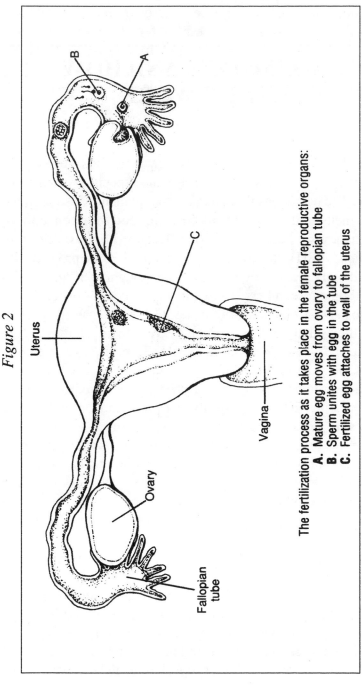

The fertilization process as it takes place in the female reproductive organs:
A. Mature egg moves from ovary to fallopian tube
B. Sperm unites with egg in the tube
C. Fertilized egg attaches to wall of the uterus

American College of Obstetricians and Gynecologists. *Your Health and the Ob/Gyn Exam.* ACOG Patient Education Pamphlet #17. Washington, DC © 1991.

6

HORMONES AND HOW
THEY WORK

Produced by glands, hormones are your body's messengers. They travel through your bloodstream to specific sites in your body. The hormones that are affected by menopause regulate your menstrual cycles, preparing your body for conception, pregnancy, and childbirth. Specifically, *follicle-stimulating hormone* (FSH) and *luteinizing hormone (LH)* are produced by the pituitary gland. Together they are thought to trigger ovulation. Some researchers believe that rises in LH during menopause may be related to hot flashes. FSH stimulates the growth of follicles that hold eggs in the ovaries. In an attempt to step up the body's estrogen production, FSH increases as the body nears menopause.

The hormones *estrogen* and *progesterone* are produced in your ovaries. Estrogen helps the endometrium, or lining of the uterus, to grow. Progesterone causes changes in the lining, which result in its being shed through menstrual periods if conception does not occur. Once ovulation becomes irregular, progesterone may not be produced, and less and less estrogen is produced by the ovaries.

It is the body's reduction in estrogen that causes the hot flashes, organ atrophy, and a myriad of other problems that surround menopause. In order to reduce these effects, many doctors now prescribe regular dosages of estrogen, referred to as *estrogen replacement therapy (ERT)*, unless there is some specific reason a woman cannot take it (see Key 19). Reasons not to take estrogen include a history of estrogen-dependent breast cancer, problems with blood clots, and severe liver disease. (When progesterone and/or testosterone

16

are taken along with estrogen, the therapy is called *hormone replacement therapy [HRT]*. In this book both terms are used to refer to the concept of taking hormones during and after menopause.)

Hormone replacement therapy originated almost a hundred years ago when a French physiologist, Dr. Charles Edouard Brown-Sequard, gave ovarian extract to women who had their ovaries removed. As discussed throughout this book, replacing estrogen during and after menopause, in many ways, gives women back the physiology they had during their reproductive years.

Fear of Endometrial Cancer Discounted

During the mid-1970s many women developed reservations about taking hormones when several studies were released showing an increased risk for endometrial cancer in women taking estrogen. However, the overall risk was actually still very low. Another factor that gained a great deal of attention during this period was that women who have high levels of estrogen naturally, such as obese women, have more endometrial cancer.

Now, however, tremendous advances have been made in administering hormones to cut down on the risk of cancer. And, most important, for most women, *lack* of estrogen causes many more problems than *taking* estrogen does (see Key 20). The bone thinning alone that results from estrogen deprivation should be enough to persuade most women to take estrogen if at all possible. In addition, estrogen reduces the risk of heart disease and stroke, prevents atrophy of internal organs, and adds to quality of life.

Moreover, there is evidence that estrogen is the reason that women live, on average, seven years longer than men. And, importantly, a recent long-term study in Great Britain showed that women who take estrogen after menopause are less likely to die of all causes than those who do not. In another study in the United States, researchers found that women who do not use estrogen are three times more likely to die of all causes than women who use estrogen.[1]

More and more benefits of estrogen replacement therapy are being discovered. A recent study by researchers at Erasmus University in the Netherlands suggests that HRT may benefit women with rheumatoid arthritis. The researchers found a two-thirds reduction in rheumatoid arthritis for women taking estrogen. The study's results suggest that one of two things may be going on. First, women with rheumatoid arthritis go into remission during pregnancy, and a similar protective measure may occur when women take estrogen. Or the hormone may suppress the inflammation that damages joints. (For a summary of the major benefits of hormone replacement therapy, see Key 20.)

---

[1]Danial R. Mishell, "Reluctance Toward Routine Estrogen Use Is Harming Our Postmenopausal Patients," *Today's Woman*, October 1990, p. 9.

7

EARLY, LATE, AND INDUCED MENOPAUSE: WHAT ARE THE FACTS?

While the average age of menopause is 51, every woman's biological clock is different. About 8 percent of women go into a natural menopause before they turn 40, and another 5 percent continue to have periods past age 53. This Key will cover both of these occurrences, which are referred to as early and late menopause, along with induced menopause, which occurs when the ovaries are surgically removed.

Early Menopause

Premature menopause may be caused by a number of medical conditions, including chromosomal abnormalities, such as Turner's syndrome, and autoimmune disorders, such as thyroiditis, diabetes mellitus, and rheumatoid arthritis. Chemotherapy and radiation can also stop ovarian function. Some women's inherited genes trigger an early shutdown of the ovaries. Smokers often begin menopause 5 to 10 years earlier than nonsmokers.

Periods may stop for other reasons than an early menopause including pregnancy, weight loss, stress, or overexercising. Some drugs taken for mental health problems can also cause periods to stop. Your doctor can diagnose a true premature menopause through blood tests. These tests check the levels of two hormones, *follicle-stimulating hormone (FSH)* and *luteinizing hormone (LH)*, that are secreted from the pituitary and that stimulate ovulation. If these levels are low, it means that you are not in menopause. If these levels are high, it means that the ovaries are not functioning properly and you are menopausal.

19

It is possible to get pregnant even if you are in a premature menopause. However, you should talk this over with your gynecologist, who may refer you to an infertility expert.

Induced Menopause

When women have their ovaries removed, the result is an instant menopause. Symptoms are usually severe, because the body is suddenly deprived of estrogen. According to Sadja Greenwood, author of *Menopause Naturally,* women whose ovaries are removed by surgery before a natural menopause run a higher risk of having a heart attack if they do not take estrogen.[1] Greenwood points out, however, that there is an advantage to an early menopause. The risk of breast cancer is reduced for women who have early menopause. Another advantage is that the risk of getting ovarian cancer is reduced because of fewer years spent ovulating.[2]

Late Menopause

If you have periods past the age of 53, you are considered to have a late menopause. You have the advantage of additional years of estrogen's protective effects on the body. As mentioned throughout this book, estrogen protects you against heart disease, osteoporosis, and atrophy of vaginal and urinary tissues. A late menopause does, however, put you at a slightly higher risk of developing ovarian cancer. Many doctors recommend that women who go into menopause late get a thorough examination of their ovaries once a year.

---

[1]Sadja Greenwood, *Menopause Naturally* (Volcano Press, 1989), p. 81.

[2]Lila E. Nachtigall and Joan Rattner Heilman, *Estrogen* (New York: Harper Perennial, 1991), p. 52.

8

SIGNS OF MENOPAUSE: CHANGES IN MENSTRUATION

Usually the first sign of menopause is a change in the regularity of periods. Menstruation may be skipped altogether or occur at irregular intervals. (You may even think you're pregnant and have a false-positive result on a urine pregnancy test. Such tests are far less reliable for women who are near menopause.) You may have a longer time between periods. Some women experience lighter and more watery periods due to a reduction in progesterone. Others have very heavy bleeding. And still others have a combination, in which they first bleed heavily for a few days and then bleed lightly. For most women, these changes are perfectly normal and nothing to worry about.

What is the normal pattern of menstruation? Most women's periods are irregular when they first start menstruating, become regular through the twenties and thirties, and then become irregular again. The interval between periods is counted from the first day of menstruation to the first day of the following period. Most periods range from 28 to 32 days. Commonly, the flow lasts three to seven days. However, some women never experience regular flow. This does not affect the time that menopause will begin.

The key word about the menstrual cycle during midlife is *change*. Your periods are different than they were previously; they may be lighter, heavier, further apart, or closer together. Some women find cramps a problem for the first time.

The Origin of Menstrual Changes During Menopause

When estrogen production decreases, ovulation is not always prompted. (Your ovaries are running out of eggs during

21

this time.) And when women stop ovulating, their bodies stop producing progesterone, causing the uterine lining to build up and shed (menstruation).

Any irregular vaginal bleeding is a warning to see a doctor right away. This is true for women of any age, but particularly after menopause. In addition, any pain or temperature that goes along with bleeding should be a warning to see a doctor immediately. Vaginal bleeding is the major sign of cervical and uterine cancer. Your doctor may prescribe progestin on a short-term basis to stop irregular bleeding.

Fibroid Tumors and Menstruation

If you have fibroid tumors in your uterus, they may also affect your periods. Fibroid tumors are growths that are usually noncancerous. As mentioned in Key 25, fibroid tumors are very common in women who are near the age of menopause. Estrogen appears to foster their growth. Women with fibroid tumors may have long or heavy periods, or both.

Keeping a Record

It will help both you and your doctor understand what is going on with your reproductive system if you keep a record of your periods. Your record should include when your periods start and end, how heavy or light the flow is, whether or not you have cramps, and, if so, how long they last. When you chart your periods over several months you may find that, indeed, your periods have changed, but they have started a new pattern.

Taking Care of Yourself During Heavy Bleeding

Heavy bleeding may be accompanied by dizziness, chills, and sweating. Unusually heavy bleeding should be evaluated by a doctor. It is important to take care of yourself during heavy periods. Be sure to get plenty of rest. You may want to cut down on physical activity. And make sure that you are getting plenty of iron and B vitamins.

9

SIGNS OF MENOPAUSE: HOT FLASHES

According to the American Medical Association, 75 percent of women experience hot flashes during menopause. Menopausal women also are particularly sensitive to heat and cold. Reports of hot flashes vary widely, ranging from constant episodes, occurring every twenty minutes or so, to one or two a year.

In the beginning, most women do not identify the heat, sweat, and palpitations they experience as hot flashes. (I thought that I was having blood sugar problems.) Here are accounts from several women describing their hot flashes.

My first hot flash occurred while I was sitting in a board meeting for my company. I looked down at my lap and noticed that beads of sweat were plopping onto my skirt. I reached my hand to my hair and realized it was soaking wet. I looked around the room and everyone else was as cool as a cucumber. I do not blush easily, but I was beet red with shame.

My husband complains because I am up and down often during the night and my side of the bed is often dripping wet. I hate to move to another room, but I feel that I may have to.

My hot flashes feel the way I imagine hell to be—I'm on fire, my heart is racing, and I'm pretty scared. Then, as quickly as they started, they are over and I am dripping wet and chilled, as if my son has left the front door open again.

Hot flashes are not harmful. Although they can be very uncomfortable, they should not be feared. Often referred to as hot flushes or vasomotor instability, hot flashes are the feeling of sudden heat bursting over the head or upper or entire body. During a hot flash the skin temperature rises as much as 7 or 8 degrees. However, the internal body temperature actually drops. Hot flashes are followed by sweating and chills.

The experience of hot flashes is different for each of us. They can last from 30 seconds to an hour, but, for most women, are over in a minute or two. They may occur frequently or rarely, at night or during the day (although they are more common in the evening). When they occur at night, they are called "night sweats." Many women feel their hot flashes coming and attempt to cool themselves off before the flashes hit. Episodes of hot flashes may last for a few months or for the rest of one's life. One-third of women have hot flashes for as long as nine years after menopause.[1]

Women who have had their ovaries removed, smoke, and are thin usually have the most severe hot flashes. In contrast, women who are overweight usually have fewer hot flashes because estrogen is manufactured in fat. Hot flashes are usually most prevalent during the first two years of menopause.

If you have hot flashes, once you know what is going on you will probably stop worrying about them. And the good news for many women is that hot flashes are greatly relieved by hormone replacement therapy.

The Origin of Hot Flashes

It is not yet known exactly why hot flashes occur. It is clear, however, that they are connected to estrogen production, because when estrogen therapy is withdrawn hot flashes reoccur. (Even men who take estrogen have hot flashes when they stop.)

---

[1]Sadja Greenwood, *Menopause Naturally* (Volcano, CA: Volcano Press, 1989), p. 26.

One theory about the origin of hot flashes is that the area of the brain that is responsible for body temperature regulation is next to the area that governs the output of hormones such as estrogen. During menopause the hormone center may throw off the adjacent temperature center. Another theory is that the hypothalamus releases a nonepinephrine substance when it does not receive estrogen.

Coping with Hot Flashes

Here are some tips for coping with hot flashes:

- Avoid anything that dilates the capillaries, such as spicy foods, caffeine, and alcohol.

- Eat frequent small meals rather than large meals.

- Drink plenty of fluids, but avoid hot drinks.

- Keep an ice pack handy to use during flashes.

- Dress in layers, so that you can shed jackets and sweaters when a flash hits. Wear natural fabrics.

- Keep the rooms you spend the most time in, including your bedroom, as cool as is comfortable.

- Stay out of the sun and hot environments.

- Be aware that emotional upset can bring on hot flashes.

- Exercise may help. A recent study conducted in Scandinavia found that women who exercise are half as likely to have hot flashes as those who do not exercise.[2]

Some women have found that vitamin E and ginseng root, a plant estrogen, help their hot flashes. Drugs sometimes prescribed other than estrogen include progestin, Bellegral, and Clonidine. Progestin is discussed throughout this book.

---

[2]M. Hammar et al., Department of Obstetrics and Gynecology, University Hospital, Linköping, Sweden.

Bellegral contains ergotamine tartrate, alkaloids of belladonna, and a sedative (phenobarbital) and is an alternative for women who cannot take estrogen. However, women with vascular disease, heart disease, high blood pressure, or glaucoma should not take Bellegral. Clonidine is a drug used primarily for high blood pressure. It also can be useful for women who cannot take estrogen.

Palpitations

You may experience a rapid heartbeat or palpitations during menopause. They may or may not occur with hot flashes. However, palpitations are thought to be caused by the same vasomotor conditions that cause hot flashes. While the palpitations are often frightening, they are not indicative of a heart problem.

10

SIGNS OF MENOPAUSE: VAGINAL CHANGES

Among the most disturbing symptoms of menopause are the marked changes in the vagina and genitals. These changes happen to all women after menopause *who do not take estrogen.* Their reproductive system returns to the condition it was in during puberty, prior to the reproductive years. In other words, without estrogen, you will essentially be housing the vagina of a five-year-old, rather than that of a midlife or older woman.

Here is what you can expect: The external genitals (vulva) and the vagina are highly responsive to estrogen and will thin out and shrink when estrogen levels decrease. Sometimes the vagina actually shortens and becomes narrower. Pubic hair also thins. Vaginal secretions become less acidic, and dryness, burning, itching, and vaginitis can result. Blood flow to the genitals decreases, and some women will actually have a narrowing of the entrance to the vagina so that intercourse will become impossible. These changes do not go away with time, but progress.

Unhappily, these changes can cause pain during sexual intercourse. As we grow older, the vaginal membrane often becomes thinner and lubrication is slower. Also, the vagina becomes far more susceptible to infection. However, the onset of vaginal dryness is not the same for everyone and some women will not experience it at all. In turn, vaginal dryness is not always caused by menopause. Some drugs may cause it, such as antihistamines, for example.

Coping with Vaginal Changes

Estrogen therapy is the best antidote for changes in the vagina. Prescription ointments such as Aci-gel can help to relieve the itchiness caused by vaginal dryness. However, Aci-gel changes the pH of the vagina, so it should not be used on a continuing basis. Lubricants can help to make sex less painful and more satisfying when the vagina is naturally dry. Types commonly available include oil-based products, such as massage oils, vitamin E oil, and cocoa butter. However, many women prefer water-based lubricants, like K-Y jelly, Koromex, and Ortho II. Two popular products available through the mail are Astroglide and Senselle.

Some doctors will prescribe estrogen cream for vaginal dryness. Estrogen cream bypasses the liver, reducing the risk of liver and gallbladder problems. However, if you are considering using estrogen cream, you should discuss the side effects with your doctor. For more information on estrogen cream, see Key 18. If you can't use estrogen cream, a testosterone cream called androgen can be applied in the same manner. However, both estrogen and androgen creams are medications to treat specific problems, and they should not be applied for lovemaking only.

Vaginal Changes and Sexuality

The bad news is that without estrogen a prepubescent, thinning vagina may become so irritated by sex that the act becomes undesirable. The good news is that sex helps to vitalize the vagina, making it more elastic and flexible, and aiding lubrication. And there is more good news. Even if you have not taken estrogen for years and your vagina has seriously atrophied, estrogen will restore it to a functioning level.

11

SIGNS OF MENOPAUSE: PREMENSTRUAL SYNDROME

As you near menopause, you may notice symptoms of premenstrual syndrome (PMS).[1] PMS is a real and often distressing set of symptoms that begin about two weeks before the start of a period. The symptoms include moodiness and depression, nervousness, irritability, fluid retention and bloating, breast swelling and tenderness, headaches, and cravings for sugar.

PMS occurs most frequently in the years prior to the beginning of menopause. It is often attributed to an imbalance in estrogen and progesterone levels. Part of the evidence for this theory is that PMS occurs during the second part of the premenstrual cycle, and it is at this time that both estrogen and progesterone are produced. During the first part of the cycle, when only estrogen is produced, PMS symptoms are absent.

At this writing, researchers are looking for other possible causes of PMS. Their research includes problems with water retention, a B vitamin deficiency, the neurotransmitter dopamine, prolactin (a pituitary hormone), and changes in carbohydrate metabolism.

Some women are so uncomfortable and have such extreme PMS symptoms that it is hard to carry out everyday activities. Others have mild symptoms, such as slight bloating. According to the classic *Merck Manual,* women who are

---

[1]Rosetta Reitz, *Menopause, a Positive Approach* (New York: Penguin, 1977), p. 17.

29

perimenopausal may have PMS symptoms during and after their periods, while younger women's symptoms usually end when their periods start.[2]

Keeping a Record

It will help both you and your doctor to understand the pattern of your PMS if you keep a record of your symptoms (as well as a record of your periods, mentioned in Key 8). Your record should include when your symptoms start and end, and the nature of your symptoms. You should also indicate whether or not you have cramps and how long they usually last, in addition to whether or not certain treatments work.

Treatment

Many women swear by vitamin B complex to minimize PMS symptoms. Specifically, some doctors suggest taking vitamin B_6 (pyridoxine). The theory behind its relationship to PMS is that women who suffer symptoms are deficient in the vitamin. Vitamin B_6 deficiency is associated with depression, bloating, and acne. Pyridoxine is also essential for hypothalamus functioning, which controls the menstrual cycle. Vitamin B_6 supplements are safe in relatively low dosages (500 mg a day), but be aware that side effects can occur with large amounts.

Natural progesterone is sometimes prescribed for PMS. It is usually prescribed to be taken from the expected time of ovulation until the beginning of the next period. Progesterone is not very convenient to use; it is taken either by suppository or by injection. Also, the suppositories must be made up by a druggist, an expensive procedure. Using natural progesterone in pill form is effective when taken in a form that dissolves *after* passage through the stomach. In addition, birth control pills and other progesterones do not relieve the symptoms of PMS.

---

[2]Robert Berkow, ed., *The Merck Manual,* 15th ed. (Rahway, NJ: Merck and Co., 1987).

Your doctor may suggest a diuretic to relieve fluid retention. Many women report that reducing bloating and edema also helps relieve other symptoms such as irritability and nervousness. However, diuretics can have serious side effects, so they should not be overused. Side effects include lethargy, excessive dryness, and potassium and sodium deficiencies.

Some doctors prescribe tranquilizers for those patients who are nervous and irritable, and antidepressants for others who are depressed. Other possible remedies include eliminating sugar, salt, processed foods, and caffeine from the diet, getting regular exercise, and taking the herbal remedy evening primrose.

Some new medications may be introduced in the near future. Presently being tested are bromocryptine, spironolactone, and antiprostaglandins.

12

SIGNS OF MENOPAUSE: URINARY INCONTINENCE

Half of all women experience urinary incontinence at some point in their lives, and a third develop a long-term problem with it. Although the condition is common, many women with the problem unnecessarily develop emotional difficulties because of their embarrassment about the condition. Some don't even talk to their doctors about it and withdraw socially because of the stress of wondering if they will have an accident while with others. In most cases, however, incontinence is treatable and can be eliminated or greatly reduced.

Urinary incontinence is most common when estrogen levels fall after childbirth and menopause. Hysterectomies can also contribute to the problem. The condition is not an inevitable part of aging. It is a common health problem that is a symptom of an underlying medical condition. It can range from slight losses of urine to frequent wetting. When wetting becomes frequent or severe enough to become a social or hygienic problem, it is time to seek advice from a doctor.

Symptoms and Types of Incontinence

Eighty percent of urine loss problems is caused by stress and urge incontinence. *Stress* incontinence, the most common type of nonintentional urine loss, typically involves losing urine with activities that put pressure on the bladder, such as lifting heavy objects, exercising, sneezing, or coughing. The underlying problem is weakness or damage to the muscles and other tissues that support the bladder and urethra, often caused by childbirth and/or reduced estrogen production during and after menopause. Such problems can be detected by physical examination.

Another major type of incontinence is *urge* incontinence, in which a loss of urine occurs whenever there is a strong desire to urinate. This type of incontinence usually involves very large accidents. Symptoms include a sudden urge to void followed by an inability to reach the toilet in time, and leaking urine whenever the urge to urinate occurs. Women may have a combination of stress and urge incontinence.

Urge incontinence is caused by a malfunctioning bladder that forces urine out of the bladder at times other than when the victim is sitting on the toilet. It can result from inflammation of the bladder or the urethra, thinning of the tissues of the urethra, and nervous system problems such as Parkinson's disease or stroke.

Other types of urinary incontinence include:
- *mixed* incontinence, a combination of stress and urge incontinence,
- *overflow* incontinence, in which urine overflows the bladder and drips out through the urethra,
- *total* incontinence, constant loss of urine,
- and *functional* incontinence, which is caused by inability to use the bathroom due to a physical limitation such as arthritis or else a lack of willingness.

Whom Should I See about This Condition? Because incontinence is a symptom of other physical problems, you should see your doctor for a complete physical. First, ask your family physician or internist if he or she is experienced in treating urinary incontinence. Specialists who treat the problem are geriatricians, urologists, and gynecologists. In addition, look in your local yellow pages to see if there is a continence clinic in your area. Physical and occupational therapists are often the best resources for effective ways to treat the problem.

Treatment Options

There are many effective treatments for urinary incontinence, including behavioral training, exercises, medicines, and surgery. In most cases, these treatments will result in curing or significantly improving the problem.

Not treating urinary incontinence can result in serious problems. For example, frequent leakage can increase the chance of skin irritation and might raise the risk of developing bedsores.

Treatment should be tailored to your particular problem or needs. In many cases, it is important to treat the underlying problem rather than the incontinence itself. Taking care of the first problem takes care of the second.

Here are details on some of the major effective treatment options for urinary incontinence:

Kegel exercises. The best-known treatment for stress incontinence is Kegel exercises, named after the doctor who developed them in 1948. The exercises involve squeezing down and contracting perineal muscles or imagining urinating and then practicing stopping immediately. The exercises should be repeated ten times at least four times a day.

Kegel exercises are very effective when done correctly, particularly if estrogen levels are high enough. In fact, they are not effective for menopausal and postmenopausal women who are not taking estrogen. The book *Staying Dry* provides excellent instruction on how to perform the exercises correctly (published by Johns Hopkins University Press).

Medications. A number of medications can be used to treat incontinence. However, they should be used carefully under a doctor's supervision because these drugs may cause side effects. The bladder actually has estrogen receptors in it. Vaginal estrogen cream can help or cure the problem.

Behavioral management techniques. These techniques include biofeedback and bladder retraining. They can help the sufferer sense bladder filling and delay voiding until on a toilet.

34

Surgery. Several types of surgery can improve or even cure incontinence that is related to a structural problem such as an abnormally shaped bladder.

Prosthetic devices. Artificial devices can replace or aid the muscles that control urine flow. However, many of these devices require surgical implantation.

Catheterization. A flexible tube known as a catheter is inserted into the urethra, and urine is collected into a container.

Electrical stimulation. The muscles around the bladder and the urethra are stimulated electrically.

Absorbent underclothing. Specially designed absorbent underclothing is available. Many of these items can be worn easily under everyday clothing and free a person from the discomfort and embarrassment of incontinence.

13

SIGNS OF MENOPAUSE: WEIGHT GAIN

For women who agree with writer Dorothy Parker that one can never be too rich or too thin, one of the unhappiest symptoms of menopause is the tendency to gain weight. In fact, in menopause the fat on the body is actually redistributed so that waists grow thicker and fat develops on the upper back and shoulders.[1] Unfortunately, estrogen replacement is not helpful with this symptom. Women on estrogen also report weight gains.[2] The latter probably occurs because of water retention and because estrogen naturally encourages development of fat tissue. Women on estrogen tend to gain weight on their breasts and hips and lose it in their waists.

Bloating and intestinal gas are also common complaints of menopause. However, the cause remains a mystery. Cutting down on salt intake and using a diuretic may help.

There are two advantages to a little extra weight after menopause. Women with more fat produce more estrogen because their body fat converts some of its androgenic hormones to estrogen. Therefore they have less trouble with hot flashes and the other symptoms of menopause. Women who are heavier also have an extra layer of fat to support their skin and, consequently, can look younger. However, the key is to have just a little plumpness and not too much. Too much weight can lead to too much estrogen and an increased risk of cancer of the uterus.

---

[1]Lila E. Nachtigall and Joan Rattner Heilman, *Estrogen* (New York: Harper Perennial, 1991), pp. 69 and 186.

[2]Ibid., p. 186.

The following tips may help with weight gain:

- As people age, the body's basic need for nutrients, such as proteins, carbohydrates, vitamins, and minerals, does not change. However, the body's need for calories **decreases**. Therefore, you will probably put on weight unless you cut back on calories and/or step up your exercise.

- To reduce bloating, cut down on salt. Your doctor may also prescribe a diuretic to take occasionally. Vitamin B_6 and cranberry juice may also help.

- You may want to consider joining a program such as Weight Watchers International, which offers a sensible, well-balanced agenda for slimming down. Equally important, the program focuses on maintaining a healthy weight. Local chapters are listed in your phone directory.

14

SIGNS OF MENOPAUSE: CHANGES IN SKIN, HAIR, AND BREASTS

Skin

Skin is the body's envelope and its largest organ. Over the years, changes take place in your skin's two layers: the outer covering, or epidermis, and the under layer, or dermis. These changes include wrinkling, age spots, sagging, dryness, and an alteration of the texture. Two important factors affect these changes—heredity and sun. In addition, estrogen depletion after menopause causes loss of fat under the skin, as well as loss of oil and moisture.

Skin Maintenance

There are four important components to maintaining healthy-looking facial skin: cleansing, moisturizing, sloughing, and protecting the skin. In addition, you may want to consider using Retin-A, described in the next section.

Cleansing. Some dermatologists recommend that older, drier skin should be washed only once a day with a soap that is not too strong. (Dove™ and Dial™ are two mild options.) Your face also should be splashed with water at least twice a day.

Moisturizing. As the skin becomes drier, moisturizing should become a daily routine. Although moisturizers cannot remove wrinkles, they do plump up the creases in the skin. The choice of moisturizers depends on skin types and preference. Dermatologists assert, however, that there is no benefit in buying expensive moisturizers. Lubriderm™ and Moisturel™

are two less expensive options. Moisturizers should be applied to slightly moist skin, which helps to trap the water and the skin's own moisture. Lotions with elastin help to fill in tiny lines and crevices.

Sloughing. Sloughing removes dead cells from the top layer of skin. Sloughing, or exfoliation, removes these cells for smoother-looking skin. Sloughing pads, such as Buf-Puf™ pads; facial scrubs that contain a rough grain such as oatmeal; or texturizing lotions, which are the least abrasive, may be used to remove dead cells.

Also, follow these tips for avoiding wrinkles:

• Drink six to eight glasses of water a day.

• Don't smoke.

• Avoid alcohol, diuretic pills, and caffeinated drinks.

• Get plenty of exercise, which nourishes the skin through increased blood flow, aids elimination of wastes through sweating, helps collagen production, and relieves stress.

• Eat foods that are good for your skin: those rich in vitamin A, D, and E, for instance.

• Never go out in the sun without using a sunscreen or wearing a cover-up.

• Get adequate rest and avoid stress.

• Do not use astringents or harsh soaps on your face.

Retin-A

If you are in search of an anti-aging skin treatment, you might want to test the tried and true product that has been found to improve aging skin. Retin-A is a 20-year-old acne treatment that reduces fine (not deep) wrinkling, stimulates blood flow, gives skin a more youthful look, and treats precancerous skin lesions.

According to Albert M. Kligman, professor of dermatology at the University of Pennsylvania, Retin-A thickens the outermost layer of the skin, causing it to look more youthful. Retin-A works by causing new skin to grow and old sundamaged skin to slough off. This effect has worked well on acne for years.

Retin-A is a chemically altered form of vitamin A; however, using unadulterated Vitamin A does not have the same effect. Users probably will find their skin becoming red and tender for the first month of use. Retin-A has to be used for the rest of your life to maintain its positive effects. Watch out for sound-alike products such as Retinyl-A that are sold over the counter and masquerade as Retin-A. Retin-A is sold only by prescription.

Hair

After menopause, many women notice an increase in facial hair and development of coarse hairs on the chin and upper lip. These changes are due to higher levels of the male hormone testosterone in relation to the level of estrogen. Unhappily, the hair on the head also often thins out. (However, baldness is very rare in women and you should consult a dermatologist if you are losing large amounts of hair.) In addition, other hair on the body grows in a more malelike pattern, making it thicker and tougher. And the hair on the head becomes drier and coarser.

Unfortunately, estrogen replacement will not greatly benefit the changes that take place in the hair on the head. However, it will help stop additional facial and body hair from developing.[1] However, the hairs that have already grown in will remain until their natural cycle is over or they are removed.

---

[1]Lila E. Nachtigall and Joan Rattner Heilman, *Estrogen* (New York: Harper Perennial, 1991), p. 147.

Facial hair can be removed with shaving, tweezing, facial bleaches, waxing, facial hair removals, or electrolysis. It is a myth that shaving makes the hair grow back thicker. Tweezing, however, can distort the root, making electrolysis difficult. Electrolysis is the most permanent treatment, but it should always be done by a professional because scarring can occur.

Here are four tips for a healthy head of hair:

1. Eat a well balanced diet.

2. Use a shampoo that is not too concentrated and drying, and use a conditioner if your hair is dry.

3. Cover your hair when you're in the sun. Sunlight dries hair.

4. Do not use heated rollers or curling irons.

Changes in Breasts

Our breasts are our mammary glands, which are designed by Nature to provide milk to newborns. They are composed of ducts, lobes, glands, fat, supporting ligaments, and underlying bone.

Breasts change throughout life, influenced by puberty, monthly menstrual cycles, pregnancy, breast feeding, birth control pills or other hormones, and, finally, menopause. During the reproductive years, breasts get lumpier, until estrogen levels are reduced and they become less lumpy, softer, and more glandular. Women with fibrocystic changes may find, as they approach menopause, that their breasts are constantly swollen and tender.[2]

Breasts also gain fibrous tissue and lose fatty tissue when estrogen levels are reduced. Lila E. Nachtigall, in her book

---

[2]Lois Janovic and Genell J. Subak-Sharpe, *Homones, the Woman's Answerbook* (New York: Fawcett Columbine, 1987), p. 206.

Estrogen, describes it this way: "The breasts shed their former thick layer of subcutaneous fat and their glandular tissue shrinks because it no longer must be ready to nourish a baby."[3] The loss of fatty tissue and elasticity results in sagging. (This is a time when being small-breasted is an advantage.) The milk-producing glands also shrink.

Breasts are extremely responsive to hormones. For example, during the reproductive years, women usually have swollen and tender breasts prior to their periods as a result of an increase in estrogen and progesterone in their systems.

All women have small amounts of breast discharge, which keep ducts in the nipple open. You may have noticed this discharge as a yellow crust. If you are on estrogen replacement therapy, you may experience increased discharge, which may be normal but must be checked. Any abnormal discharge, such as that containing blood, milk, pus, or yellow liquid, should be checked by a doctor.

---

[3]Lila E. Nachtigall and Joan Rattner Heilman, *Estrogen* (New York: Harper Perennial, 1991).

15

SIGNS OF MENOPAUSE: SLEEP CHANGES

Menopause affects the ability to get a good night's sleep. In fact, after hot flashes, the inability to sleep at night (insomnia) is the second most frequent menopause-related complaint that women make to their doctors.[1] Most of the literature on menopause attributes sleep problems to an inability to fall asleep after severe hot flashes. But as any of us who have experienced menopause-related insomnia know, there is much more to it than that. Even when I have been on estrogen and progestin, my sleeplessness consistently has occurred several days before withdrawal bleeding. And hot flashes did not accompany my periods of wakefulness. Many other women have had similar experiences. Lila E. Nachtigall and Joan Rattner Heilman, in the excellent book *Estrogen*, assert that menopausal sleeplessness is caused by hypothalamic disturbances that overstimulate the central nervous system.

Menopause is not the only cause of sleep problems in midlife and beyond. Sleep patterns change for both men and women. In short, after the middle years, it takes longer to get to sleep, less time is spent in deep sleep (the most restorative cycle of sleep), and sleep is easily disturbed. Researchers feel that the changes in sleep patterns as people age are related to changes in hormone levels.

Sleep Disorders

Most of us think that men are the snorers, keeping their sleepless wives awake all night as they rattle the bed-

---

[1]Lila E. Nachtigall and Joan Rattner Heilman, *Estrogen* (New York: Harper Perennial, 1991), p. 65.

room windows. And, on average, this is true—up to about the age of 50. The results of a recent study in Italy demonstrate that chronic snoring among men increases significantly with age and that most women do not snore—until age 50. Then researchers found a steady increase in snoring among women. The change is caused by a depletion in estrogen, which protects women from having difficulty in breathing or from snoring during sleep.

In addition to *snoring*, other breathing problems occur more frequently during sleep as people grow older. Some problems can lead to serious medical conditions. For example, sleep *apnea*, described below, causes fatigue, raises blood pressure (particularly for people who snore), raises the risk of stroke, and can cause cardiac arrhythmia.

Insomnia is disturbing at any age. It is the most common sleep problem and is usually a symptom of another problem. Insomnia means taking a long time to fall asleep (more than a half-hour or 45 minutes), waking up many times each night, or waking up early and not being able to get back to sleep.

Sleep apnea is a problem where breathing stops for up to 2 minutes and the person struggles to breathe, even though unaware of it. Two clues are daytime sleepiness and loud snoring. Techniques are available to help people with this problem, including devices to keep people off their backs and an approach called continuous positive airway pressure, in which the individual wears a mask that aids breathing. Ask your doctor for a referral to an occupational therapist or sleep specialist who can recommend the best devices and techniques for your particular problem.

Coping with Sleep Problems

Paradoxically, many of the medications, including tranquilizers and antidepressants, that are prescribed for insomnia and other sleep problems end up exacerbating the situation. When people who take these drugs for a while try to get a good night's sleep without them, they have what is called a rebound effect, which often causes a worse case of insomnia than the one they started with. And even though these medications do knock people out, they provide a different type of sleep than the restorative deep sleep that individuals get naturally. A good rule of thumb is to take these medications only occasionally, and only when not taking them poses a health risk.

One of the best rules for getting a good night's sleep is not to fight it. To get to sleep you have to relax. Doctors suggest that if you do not fall asleep after a half hour, get out of bed and do something to relax—take a hot bath, read poetry, or watch a soothing video. The point is to avoid doing anything too stimulating. Don't stay in bed and toss and turn where you can get situational insomnia, which means that you associate your bed with sleeplessness. These tips for getting a good night's sleep are adapted from the National Institutes on Health:

- *Exercise* daily to relieve restless legs, which are muscle twitches that can cause brief arousals from sleep, and tensions that disturb sleep.
- Try to go to bed at the *same time* each night and get up at the same time each day, regardless of the time you went to sleep.
- *Do not eat* for two hours before you go to sleep.
- Just before going to bed, drink a glass of *warm milk*, which contains a sleep-promoting amino acid.
- Many people find that a *hot bath* before retiring brings on yawns and heavy lids.
- To adjust your internal sleep clock, try to get some exposure to *natural light* in the afternoon each day.
- Avoid drinking *caffeinated* beverages (coffee, tea, chocolate, soft drinks such as cola) after 4:00 P.M. A stimulant, caffeine can keep you awake. Monosodium glutamate (MSG), a seasoning used in some Chinese cooking, can have the same effect.

- Don't drink *alcohol* or *smoke cigarettes* to help you sleep. Although many people use alcohol to sleep, it actually disturbs the sleep process, and too much of it can cause insomnia. Nicotine in cigarettes is a stimulant.
- Develop a bedtime *routine*. Do the same things each night to tell your body that it's time to run down. Some people watch the evening news, read a book, or soak in a warm bath.
- Use your bedroom *only* for sleeping. After turning off the light, give yourself about 15 minutes of trying to fall asleep. If you are still awake, or if you lose your drowsiness, get up and go into another room until you feel sleepy again.
- Try using aids such as specially shaped *pillows* or *footboards* to maintain good posture while sleeping.
- Try out some of the *relaxation techniques* discussed in Key 42. Also try visualizing a peaceful place or a black wall, and concentrate on listening to your breathing.
- Try to do *restful, peaceful things* before you go to sleep. Don't attempt to work out *problems* while you are trying to nod off.
- Don't go to bed *earlier*. It will spread out sleep and won't be satisfying.

In addition, a comfortable bed with a good, comfortable, firm mattress is important. The bed should support the spine and not sag in the middle. You may want to try out a heated waterbed, but try it before you buy it. These beds are expensive and some people swear by them, while others—and this could be you—can't stand them. An electric blanket or mattress pad may also be helpful.

When to see a doctor. If you are so tired during the day that you cannot function normally and this condition lasts for two or three weeks, you should see your family doctor or a sleep disorder specialist.

16

SIGNS OF MENOPAUSE: MOOD CHANGES

An early sign of menopause is moods that swing back and forth along with estrogen levels. These undulating emotions often come at a time when many other pivotal changes are also happening in life—that is, the kids are leaving home, mom and dad are growing frail, and/or other physical problems are popping up. For many women this is also a time when they begin to face their aging and ultimate mortality. Here is the story of one woman who started her menopause at age 40:

> *Sally was having severe migraines and went from doctor to chiropractor to herbalist for help. Finally an aunt figured out her problem during a family reunion. Sally had looked forward to the get-together, which was taking place in the next state, but once she arrived at her aunt's house, she could not stop weeping. And when she wasn't shedding tears, she was coping with blinding headaches. Finally, not unlike Mrs. Threadgoode to Evelyn in* Fried Green Tomatoes at the Whistle Stop Cafe, *her aunt said, "Dear, you're in menopause. You go see your doctor as soon as you get home." And she did. When her hormone tests came back indicating she was deep in menopause, no one was more surprised than her doctor, who had tied her tubes a couple of months earlier!*

The symptoms of the mood swings that occur during this time in life are not pleasant and include *anxiety*, *anger*, *depression*, *headaches*, *fatigue*, and *nervousness*. There is reason to take heart, however. According to leading gynecologist and menopause expert Dr. Lila Nachtigall, these emotions are early symptoms that usually fade in under a year.[1]

You will find that *mood swings* are greatly improved by taking estrogen. This fact has been proven by clinical studies done by Professor Barbara Sherwin at McGill University. Some women also find relief by taking testosterone. Others swear by B complex vitamins, often referred to as antistress vitamins. Calcium and vitamin C also are often recommended for calming frazzled nerves. A small number of women need the help of tranquilizers or antidepressants to get through this period. However, such mood-altering drugs are usually not a long-term option. They should be used only during this transition time when raging hormones are truly upsetting emotional equilibrium.

If you are not in *therapy*, this is a good time to consider short-term help as a way of looking at the pros and cons of this midlife passage. I had a very difficult time facing my shrinking years and letting go of the prospects of ever having a child. I found a very focused, good psychotherapist who helped me close some doors that I was trying to keep open against strong winds and open other doors that I was keeping shut out of fear. I am grateful for the help in adjusting to this time and place in my life.

---

[1]Lila E. Nachtigall and Joan Rattner Heilman, *Estrogen* (New York: Harper Perennial, 1991), p. 67.

17

SIGNS OF MENOPAUSE: OSTEOPOROSIS

Osteoporosis, or porous bone, is a menopause-related condition in which bone mass decreases, causing bones to fracture easily. One-third to one-half of all postmenopausal women have this bone-wasting disease.

Osteoporosis is so closely linked to menopause that it is the *number of years past your menopause*, not your chronological age, that indicates the strength of bones. The protection of estrogen is present up to the time of menopause, when its levels begin to decrease.

Osteoporosis causes 1.3 million fractures each year to people over age 45. Twelve to 20 percent of people with hip fracture die within a year after the fracture. However, researchers agree that osteoporosis is *highly preventable* through taking estrogen, exercising regularly, and taking in adequate calcium.

What Makes Up Bones?

In order to understand how osteoporosis affects bone, it is useful to understand what bones are made of. Calcium and protein are the building blocks of bone. Compact bone refers to the outside structure and is solid and hard. Spongy bone is filled with holes and is on the inside of all bones. Osteoporosis first hits those parts of the body that have a lot of spongy bone, such as the spine, the hip, and the wrist. As the disease progresses, the wall of compact bone becomes thin and the holes in the spongy bone become larger.

Many people think of bones as hard and inert. However, they are constantly changing. In a process referred to as *remodeling*, two types of cells within the bones break down old bone and make new bone. Up until age 35, bone is made faster than it is broken down. Then after age 35, the reverse is true, causing a loss of bone mass. The loss is part of the natural aging process and does not necessarily result in problems. It is when the loss is too rapid that osteoporosis can occur, weakening the bones to the point that they break easily.

It is also useful to remember that bones have purposes other than forming the body's infrastructure. They are the body's storehouse of calcium, and they are constantly releasing and resorbing the mineral in response to hormone signals. For this reason, adequate calcium intake is important to maintaining strong bones.

There are two types of osteoporosis classified according to the type of resorption and formation of bone that takes place:

1. Type I (or *high turnover*) osteoporosis results when bone resorption is too high and there is a disproportionate loss of spongy bone. It tends to result in spinal or forearm fractures.

2. In Type II (or *low turnover*) osteoporosis, both inner and outer bone is lost because of lack of formation. It tends to cause fractures in the vertebrae, hip, pelvis, and long bones.

Estrogen and Your Bones

Numerous studies, an expert panel convened by the National Institutes of Health, and the American Medical Association have pinpointed estrogen as the best deterrent to osteoporosis in women. For example, a ten-year study at Goldwater Memorial Hospital in New York found that women who take estrogen after menopause do not develop osteoporosis, while those who do not take it do. Estrogen in minimum doses of 0.625 mg a day will prevent osteoporosis from developing. However, it must be started within three years after your last menstrual period.

Drugs and Osteoporosis

Drugs can contribute to or help prevent osteoporosis. For example, fluoridation of water appears to help maintain strong bones, as well as strong teeth. In fact, doctors sometimes prescribe fluoride supplements to treat osteoporosis. On the other hand, cortisone, which is useful in treating inflammation, promotes bone loss. Other drugs that contribute to bone loss are diuretics, aluminum-containing antacids, thyroid supplements, and anticonvulsant drugs. (For more information on drugs that can help prevent osteoporosis see the section that follows on treatment.)

Who Develops Osteoporosis?

If you are a woman and are thin, small-boned, white, and postmenopausal, you are at high risk for developing osteoporosis. There are a number of identifiable factors for developing osteoporosis:

Age. The likelihood of developing osteoporosis increases with age.

Sex. Women are six to eight times more likely to develop the condition than men.

Early or surgical menopause. A sudden drop in estrogen is associated with an increased risk for osteoporosis. Women who experience menopause before age 45 are particularly likely to develop osteoporosis.

Race. Whites are more likely to develop the condition than blacks. In fact, on average, blacks have 10 percent more bone mass than whites.

Low calcium intake.

Lack of weight-bearing exercise.

Being underweight.

A family history of the condition.

Smoking cigarettes.

Excessive use of cortisone type drugs such as prednisone.

Symptoms

Unfortunately, osteoporosis usually does not show up until significant bone loss has taken place. It may go undetected until one day you realize that your waist is thicker and you can't diet the excess off or you have lost an inch or two in height. These are permanent changes caused by collapsed vertebrae in the spine. Collapsed vertebrae are also sometimes felt as severe back pain or result in a curvature of the back, called "dowager's hump."

Diagnosis

Early detection of osteoporosis is important to cut down on advancing bone loss. However, as mentioned previously, it is usually very hard to detect problems until a significant amount of damage has occurred. Bone loss cannot be determined by X-ray until 30 percent of bone density has been lost. Two common techniques used to get more accurate readings are photon absorptiometry, which is used to measure bone density, and computerized tomography (CT), which uses X-rays to create a three-dimensional image.

Prevention

Dr. Lawrence Shulman, head of the National Institute on Arthritis, Musculoskeletal, and Skin Disease, emphasizes that prevention is the key to decreasing the statistics on osteoporosis. "We have to be sure that we build up as much bone as possible in early life and that we lose as little as possible after mid-life," says Shulman. "We need to put some bone reserves in the bank." To help build strong bones, in addition to taking estrogen, follow these guidelines:

• Eat a balanced diet rich in calcium (see Key 40).
• Exercise regularly (see Key 39).
• Limit alcohol intake.
• Don't smoke.

Treatment

A major treatment for women is estrogen therapy, which, as mentioned, slows bone loss and prevents fractures. It is important to start taking estrogen *as soon as menopause begins*. However, estrogen therapy is still effective if begun as late as ten to fifteen years after menopause. It must be continued in order to prevent bone loss.

You also should take 1,200 to 1,500 milligrams of calcium a day, equivalent to four or five eight-ounce glasses of milk.

Other sources of calcium are yogurt, cheese, salmon, canned sardines, oysters, shrimp, dried beans, and dark green vegetables. Because calcium supplements are often not absorbed sufficiently, eating calcium-rich foods is preferable to taking calcium tablets. However, if you cannot tolerate dairy products and must take calcium supplements, calcium citrate appears to be the best supplement. (See Key 40 for more information on calcium and diet.) If you take antacids to add calcium to your diet, stay away from those that contain aluminum derivatives, because they cause loss of calcium from the body.

Excessive dietary fat and protein in the diet should be avoided, as they interfere with calcium absorption. In addition, vitamin D is necessary for calcium absorption. Normal healthy adults who are outdoors every day for about 30 minutes do not need to take vitamin D supplements.[1] However, individuals who are not, should take 400 to 800 IUs (international units) a day.

Studies have shown that lack of exercise results in bone loss. To slow down osteoporosis, the National Institutes on Health recommends a program of moderate weight-bearing exercise three to four hours a week, such as brisk walking, running, tennis, or aerobic dance. Nonweight-bearing exercise such as swimming is not as effective.

Finally, three major drugs are used to treat osteoporosis. Calcitonin injections and etridonate (Didronel™) have been found to be effective at retarding loss of bone mass and are used to treat Type I osteoporosis.[2] Calcitonin also provides pain relief. Sodium fluoride has been used to stimulate bone growth and is used to treat Type II osteoporosis. If you have significant bone loss you may want to ask your doctor about these chemicals.

---

[1]Karyn Holm and Jane Walker, *Geriatric Nursing*, May/June 1990, pp. 141–142.
[2]Angelo A. Licata, "Therapies for Symptomatic Primary Osteoporosis," *Geriatrics*, November 1991, pp. 62–67.

18

HORMONE REPLACEMENT THERAPY (HRT)

The standard approach to hormone replacement therapy is to take both estrogen and progesterone. Estrogen may be taken in pill form or by skin patch, vaginal creams, and injections. *Conjugated estrogen* in pill form (Premarin™) is prescribed most frequently. The minimal effective dosage is 0.625 mg. However, a higher dosage may be required. The disadvantage of taking estrogen in tablet form is that relatively high dosages are required because the liver absorbs much of the hormone. Progesterone is also given in tablet form.

Estrogen *creams* and *patches* are also available. Topical estrogen creams can be applied directly to the vagina and are effective for treating vaginal and urinary symptoms. A small amount of the estrogen gets into the bloodstream. If estrogen cream is used for vaginal treatment only, your doctor will probably require that you use it every day for a while and then two or three times a week indefinitely.

Estrogen patches contain 0.05 mg of estrogen, which is absorbed through the skin. The patches (Estraderm™) are placed on the lower abdomen or hip and must be changed twice a week. The advantage of the patch over the tablet form is that the hormone is released into the bloodstream in a low steady dosage, while the pills deliver a larger dosage in one large burst. Estrogen delivered by patch also bypasses the liver. However, the patches may cause skin irritation.

A good rule of thumb for taking estrogen has been suggested by Dr. Charles Dafoe, a Denver, Colorado, gynecologist. He advises that, first, women should take the minimal dosage that works for them—in other words, the smallest dosage that will relieve such menopausal symptoms as mood swings and hot flashes. Second, they should adjust their medication every five years to see if a lower dosage would be effective. However, a doctor should check your blood levels. If they are too low, the dosage is not protecting you from osteoporosis.

HRT Must Be Taken with Food

Some doctors feel that estrogen and progesterone must be taken with some fat in order to be absorbed by the body. However, you do not need to take them with an entire meal. Any small amount of food with adequate fat, such as a glass of 1 percent milk, half a banana, or cheese and crackers will do.

Side Effects

Although the doses used for hormone therapy are relatively low and side effects are not common, you may experience any of the following symptoms for a couple of months: salt and water retention causing bloating, weight gain, breast swelling and tenderness, headaches, nausea, vomiting, dizziness, and vaginal infections. These side effects should go away, or you and your doctor should discuss changing your dosage.

How Long Should I Take Estrogen?

In the past, many doctors have recommended stopping HRT after a few years. However, this is no longer the standard, because it is now widely understood that the long-term benefits of estrogen can increase the quality of life and cut down on the risk of a number of chronic and potentially fatal health conditions.

How to Take Estrogen

As of this writing, there are four major methods for taking estrogen and progesterone. However, many advances are being made in hormone replacement therapy, so it is important to discuss your particular regimen with your doctor at least once a year at the time that you have your annual gynecological exam.

Testosterone may be added to estrogen and progesterone to help alleviate symptoms. It is your job to work out with your doctor the method that works best for you. You may have to try several different regimens, including some not listed here, before you hit on the one that works best. With almost all of these methods, unless you have had your uterus removed, you can expect some bleeding, referred to as withdrawal bleeding.

Mimicking the menstrual cycle. With this method you take estrogen every day of the month and progestin for 12 to 14 days. Potential side effects include irritability, tiredness, breast tenderness, slight bleeding, and headaches.

Five to nine days without hormones. This method involves going off all hormones for 5 to 9 days. You take estrogen for 21 to 25 days only in combination with progestin for 7 to 12 of those days. This method was developed to lessen the stimulation of the uterus.

Continuous HRT. This method protects against the risk of cancerous cells developing in the uterus by blocking growth of the uterine lining. You take estrogen and a low dose of progestin daily. Side effects are limited and menstrual cycles will eventually be minimal.

Taking estrogen alone. This method is for women who have had a hysterectomy. Estrogen alone is taken daily. Some doctors consider this method to be outmoded and feel that even women without a uterus should take progesterone along with estrogen, because it more naturally mimics nature. In other words, during the years when your body was producing estrogen, it was also producing progesterone.

19

WHEN NOT TO TAKE HRT

In the past, the standard of treatment for prescribing HRT has been conservative. Consequently many women who should have been taking hormones did not get them. The result was osteoporosis, heart disease, thinning tissues, and related conditions.

Now many researchers and doctors are changing their thinking on this matter. The reason is that, as discussed throughout this book, in most cases, the risks of *not* taking estrogen are greater than the risks of *taking* it.

On the other hand, you may be one of the women who should absolutely not take estrogen because you have a specific condition that it would aggravate. According to the *Merck Manual,* used by physicians for diagnosis and therapy, the conditions that prohibit taking estrogen are:

- a history of estrogen-dependent tumors of the breast or lining of the uterus.

- a history of problems with blood clots (thrombophlebitis or thromboembolism).

- severe liver disease.

In addition, if you have any of the following problems, you and your doctor should be especially careful in watching your estrogen replacement therapy: fibroid tumors, unscheduled bleeding, obesity, diabetes, hypertension, and gallbladder disease.

If you cannot take estrogen you should be sure to:

- eat a balanced diet that is high in calcium.

- get plenty of weight-bearing exercise.

- not smoke.

- have regular complete medical checkups.

Moreover, taking a calcium supplement to guard against osteoporosis becomes even more important (see Key 17). Medications such as calcitonin can help ward off the effects of osteoporosis. Others, such as Clonidine or Catapres, can provide relief from hot flashes. You should also use a vaginal lubricant (see Key 10).

20

THE PROS AND CONS OF ESTROGEN—A SUMMARY

Estrogen has been called the great normalizer because, in many ways, it gives women back the physiology they had during their reproductive years. No, if you're in your forties, you're not going to wake up one day and look 17 (or 27, or even 37). But a number of wonderful things will happen. If you have been experiencing hot flashes, they will be greatly reduced. If you have been tossing and turning at night, you finally will be able to sleep soundly. If your vagina is dry and your libido is low, moisture will return and your desire for sex will come back.

And, perhaps most important, your chances of developing the following chronic and/or potentially fatal conditions will be greatly decreased: osteoporosis, heart disease, stroke, urinary incontinence (which is surprisingly common), and related health problems.

On the next page, you will find a summary of the pros and cons of taking estrogen. I suspect that when you add them up, it will be very clear that the pros outweigh the cons, unless there is a specific reason why you cannot take estrogen (see Key 19).

ESTROGEN—THE GREAT NORMALIZER

	Pros		Cons
Overall health	Women who do <u>not</u> take estrogen are three times more likely to die of all causes.	*Hypertension*	One in 20 women have a rise in blood pressure. By using estrogen vaginal cream or the transdermal skin patch in place of a tablet, the problem can be side-stepped.
Coronary heart disease	Reduces risk 44 to 50 percent.		
Strokes	Reduces risk 30 percent or more.	*Gallstones*	Affects bile in the liver. By using estrogen vaginal cream or the transdermal skin patch in place of a tablet, the problem can be side-stepped.
Bone thinning (osteoporosis)	Significant reduction in risk.		
Vagina and vulva	Restored to normal.		
Mood swings	Greatly reduced.	*Fibroids*	Fibroid tumors can proliferate.
Hot flashes	Greatly reduced.		
Sexual intercourse	Restores comfort and, therefore, pleasure. Restores libido.	*Expense*	Hormone replacement therapy has a high annual cost and must be taken for the remaining years of life to maintain benefits.
Skin	Moisture restored and firmer.		
Muscles	Firmer and stronger.		**Concerns**
Hair	Stronger.		
Breasts	Firmer.	*Breast cancer*	Although it does not appear to cause breast cancer, estrogen may promote the growth of preexisting tumors. Some studies have shown it to be protective against breast cancer. Others have found it to be a risk for women who take it for a long time.
Arthritis	Some studies have shown that estrogen relieves arthritic pain and reduces the incidence of rheumatoid arthritis.		
Snoring	Eliminated.	*Uterine cancer*	No increased risk when used with progesterone. It may, however, make already existing cancers grow faster.
Sleep problems	Greatly reduced.		

Sources

Lila E. Nachtigall and Joan Rattner Heilman, *Estrogen* (New York: Harper Perennial, 1991).
Council on Scientific Affairs, "Estrogen Replacement in the Menopause," *Journal of the American Medical Association*, Jan. 21, 1983, vol. 249.
American Cancer Society (ACS), *Cancer Facts and Figures,* ACS, 1992.
Robert Berkow, ed., *The Merck Manual,* 15th ed., Merck, Sharpe and Doehme Research Laboratories, 1987.
Morton A. Stenchever and George Aagaard, *Caring for the Older Woman*, Elsevier, 1991.
Dr. Lawrence Scrima, Rose Sleep Disorders Center, Denver, CO.

21

AMERICAN MEDICAL ASSOCIATION GUIDELINES FOR ESTROGEN REPLACEMENT THERAPY

In January 1983 the American Medical Association published guidelines for practicing physicians in regard to estrogen use and postmenopausal women.[1] Although the report appeared some time ago, the guidelines provide important facts about estrogen's benefits and risks. Specifically, the report states that estrogen is effective in the treatment or prevention of osteoporosis, atrophy of the urogenital system, hot flashes, and heart disease. Highlights from the report are summarized in this key.

Benefits of Estrogen Therapy

The AMA lists four specific instances where women will benefit from taking estrogen:

Osteoporosis. The report states that estrogen therapy reduces the incidence of spinal, hip, and other bone fractures. Importantly, it states: "Treatment is most effective when given before significant bone loss has occurred and has been shown to delay bone loss for at least eight years; information on the effects of longer use is not available. When estrogen treatment is withdrawn, bone loss resumes."

Genitourinary atrophy. Estrogen relieves symptoms caused by atrophy of tissues in the female reproductive tract and

---

[1]Council on Scientific Affairs, "Estrogen Replacement in the Menopause," *Journal of the American Medical Association*, Jan. 21, 1983, vol. 249, no. 3.

urinary system. Specifically, the report states that: "Both oral and topical preparations are effective."

Vasomotor flushes. Estrogen has a demonstrable and significant effect in reducing the intensity and number of hot flashes. Symptoms reappear after withdrawal of the hormone.

Coronary artery disease. The report points out that until menopause occurs, women have a lower incidence of coronary artery disease than men. After menopause, their risk equals that of men. Taking estrogen improves women's serum high-density lipoprotein (HDL) level (known as the "good" cholesterol), thus giving them back the benefit they had prior to menopause.

Risks of Estrogen Therapy
The AMA report lists these risks of taking estrogen:

Endometrial cancer. The report points out that studies of estrogen and endometrial cancer are conflicting. They conclude that:
1. estrogen administration does increase significantly the incidence of endometrial cancer
2. it does not increase mortality of the disease.

(It's important to remember that this report came out before combining estrogen and progesterone became common. Progesterone was introduced to prevent the risk of endometrial cancer.)

Uterine bleeding. Uterine bleeding is a common complication of estrogen and should always be followed diligently because of the possibility of uterine malignancy.

Other adverse effects. Fluid retention, breast enlargement, and growth of preexisting uterine myomas (tumors) can occur. According to the report, *"Studies attempting to identify a possible relationship between menopausal estrogen therapy and breast cancer have not produced significant evidence of such a link."*

Specific Recommendations of the AMA

The AMA emphasizes the following points in regard to taking estrogen:[2]

- Estrogen should be used in the smallest effective dosage and for the shortest period that satisfies therapeutic need. (Medical thinking in regard to the latter point now encourages women to continue to use HRT for the postmenopausal years to prevent osteoporosis and protect against heart disease.)

- Estrogens are effective in the treatment or prevention of hot flashes, atrophy of the urogenital system, osteoporosis, and heart disease.

- Any vaginal bleeding in the postmenopausal patient should be investigated promptly.

- Yearly monitoring of women taking estrogen should be performed by their doctors.

- Women with estrogen-dependent neoplasms of the breast or a history of such lesions should not take estrogen.

---

[2] The AMA's guideline recommending cyclic administration of estrogen has been omitted to prevent confusion by those women who are on continuous hormone therapy.

22

NONPRESCRIPTION APPROACHES

This Key covers nonprescription approaches to alleviating the symptoms of menopause. They are particularly important for women who cannot take estrogen.

Vitamin E. Many women swear by vitamin E to relieve hot flashes. Dr. Lila E. Nachtigall recommends starting with 400 units twice a day and doubling the dose if that doesn't work.[1] Sources for vitamin E are wheat germ, whole grains, vegetable oils, eggs, green vegetables, beans, peas, peanuts, walnuts, filberts, and almonds.

B, C, and Other Vitamins. Many women believe that there are benefits from taking vitamins B and C, on a regular basis, although no studies have been done that can document that fact. Both vitamins also promote healthy skin, and many believe that vitamin C is calming. B vitamins can be found in whole grains, brewer's yeast, lean meats, organ meats, poultry, fish, dried beans, and peas. Vitamin C can be found in citrus fruits and juices, broccoli, strawberries, cantaloupe, tomatoes, cabbage, green peppers, potatoes, green leafy vegetables, and sprouts.

Calcium. Not only is calcium necessary to combat osteoporosis, but it is also calming. Many women use it to fall asleep.

---

[1]Lila E. Nachtigall and Joan Rattner Heilman, *Estrogen* (New York: HarperPerennial, 1991), p. 75.

Herbs and Roots. Some women have tried using herbs and roots with moderate to complete success. However, a word of caution is in order. Herbs and roots can be dangerous. *Never take them without advice from someone with a lot of experience*, preferably a licensed physician. Herbs commonly used for menopause are ginseng and black cohosh, which actually contain estrogen. In fact, if you are not supposed to take estrogen replacement therapy, *stay away from these two.* Other herbs and roots often used include licorice root, golden seal, and valerian root. An excellent source of finding out about herbs to treat menopause is *Ourselves, Growing Older* by the Boston Women's Health Book Collective.

23

PELVIC RELAXATION

About half of all women eventually experience an unpleasant relaxation or sagging of muscles and organs in the pelvic area after menopause. The sagging, or prolapse, is caused by a weakening of the tissues that normally support the bladder, urethra, rectum, and/or uterus.

Pelvic relaxation can be uncomfortable and embarrassing. Symptoms range from mild to severe. Some women are actually symptom free. Others with advanced conditions experience a feeling that their organs are literally falling out of their body. And, indeed, organs can actually protrude through the floor of the pelvis. There are measures, such as performing Kegel exercises (see Key 12) and taking estrogen, that can cut down on the severity of pelvic relaxation. However, they cannot totally cure it.

Causes of Pelvic Relaxation

Prolapse is usually the result of childbirth and reduced estrogen. However, the victim frequently is not aware of it until menopause, when symptoms grow worse. Any prolonged activity that causes stress on the pelvic muscles, such as heavy lifting and straining at the toilet, can contribute to the problem.

Symptoms

As discussed previously, pelvic relaxation can lead to urinary incontinence (see Key 12 for a list of symptoms). Some women notice prolapse as a loss of sensation during sexual intercourse. Sometimes, protruding organs can be felt by inserting a finger in the rectum or vagina, or they can be seen bulging through the vagina.

Types of Prolapse

The following describes the major types of pelvic relaxation:

Cystocele. This is a condition where the bladder extrudes into the vaginal canal. It may be difficult to completely empty the bladder, and infections may develop.

Prolapsed uterus. The uterus sags into the vaginal canal. In more advanced stages, the uterus may be seen outside the vagina. The bladder, rectum, or urethra may also be prolapsed.

Urethrocele. This is a condition where the urethra, the tube that connects the bladder to the urinary opening, protrudes into the vaginal wall.

Rectocele. The rectum protrudes into the back wall of the vagina. Constipation may result.

Relaxation of the vagina. In this condition, a complete prolapse may not be present, but the muscles that keep the vagina snug have relaxed.

Treatment

Once prolapse has occurred, estrogen therapy cannot cure it. It can, however, cut down on the thinning and loss of elasticity of muscles. Surgery may be required to strengthen and prop up the bladder, uterus, and/or rectum. Sometimes a hysterectomy is also required (see below). The vagina can be tightened surgically.

If surgery cannot be performed, a *pessary* can be used. A pessary is a plastic or rubber appliance that fits in the vagina and holds the uterus, bladder, and other organs in place. Unfortunately, pessaries are not great long-term options, as they can be irritating and cause discharges, they can interfere with sexual intercourse, and they must be taken out and cleaned at least once a week.

Avoiding Hysterectomy for a Prolapsed Uterus

The second most common reason for performing hysterectomies, in addition to fibroid tumors, is a prolapsed uterus. However, unless a hysterectomy is accompanied by a reconstructive propping up of other organs, it can cause the prolapse of the vagina, bladder, or bowel. Since the latter procedure is complicated, it should only be done by surgeons who successfully perform it often.

24

VAGINITIS AND OTHER INFECTIONS

Reduction in estrogen levels can result in the discomfort of frequent vaginal and urinary infections. However, most of that discomfort can be prevented by taking estrogen in one of its available forms.

Vaginal infections are the result of the weakness of the vaginal lining and a change from an acidic to an alkaline level, which occur when estrogen is depleted. In turn, the weakness and alkaline pH of the vagina result in a susceptibility to irritation and infection. Urinary infections result from weakness in the urethra and bladder, which are located close to the vagina, allowing for easy transmission of infection from the vaginal area.

If you have reoccurring vaginal and/or urinary infections, and you are on HRT, ask your doctor about increasing your dosage of estrogen or about using vaginal estrogen cream in addition to it. Estrogen cream will not only help to plump up your tissues and provide moisture, but will also create a more acidic pH. (The lubricant Replens™ also helps to restore the vagina to a more acidic level.)

Different forms of vaginal infection can occur. Two major types are yeast and bacterial infections. Yeast infections occur when natural yeast, which always inhabit the vagina, gets out of control. The result is a painful itching and burning sensation. Bacterial infections can result from sexual intercourse or improper wiping of the rectum (women should always wipe from the front to the back to avoid infection).

Here are some tips that can help you cut down on vaginal and related infections: .

- As a general rule avoid using *douches*, which will only help to make dry tissue drier.

- Use a *lubricant* such as Astroglide™ during sexual intercourse.

- Use a moisturizer for the vagina, such as Replens™, two or three times a week.

- Wear *cotton* underpants and avoid wearing synthetics near the skin.

- Wear *loose-fitting* clothing.

- Wear *protection* if having sexual intercourse with anyone who is not a steady partner.

- Antibiotics and penicillin can result in infections. Your doctor may give you a prescription for a *medication* to take along with them to prevent infection.

- *Acidophilus* in yogurt, acidophilus milk, or acidophilus tablets help ward off infection. Many of the commercial yogurts will not work, however, as they do not have acidophilus.

- Drink at least eight glasses of *water* a day to keep your urine diluted.

- Be sure to empty your *bladder* every few hours. Urine sitting in the bladder too long can become a breeding ground for infection.

Treatment

Acidophilus products will help the treatment of vaginal yeast infections, as well as working to prevent them. In addition, two popular and effective drugs, Gyne-Lotrimin™

and Monistat™, have been available over the counter for some time now. But any product containing miconazole and related chemicals is equally effective. These drugs should be used only if you are sure you have a yeast infection and not another condition.

Vaginal infections caused by bacteria are often treated with Flagyl™ (metronidazole). This drug, however, should not be taken if you are pregnant. Many women find help for bacterial infections from a vinegar douche of one to two tablespoons in a quart of water. Others find that drinking cranberry juice and taking vitamin C provide some relief from urinary infections. Your doctor will take a culture for testing if your vaginal infections persist. A drug called Mandelamine™ is sometimes prescribed.

25

FIBROID TUMORS OF
THE UTERUS

The term *fibroid tumor* frightens many women. However, the good news is that tumors are not synonymous with cancer. They are swellings or growths that can be cancerous or noncancerous. And in more than 9 out of 10 cases, fibroid tumors are benign. In other words, they are rarely death warrants. (Noncancerous tumors are referred to as *benign*, and *malignant* is used to describe cancerous tumors.)

Fibroid tumors are growths in the muscle of the uterine wall (called the *myometrium*). These growths are also called *myomas* or *leiomyomas*. Contrary to what you would expect from the name *fibroid*, myomas are made up not of fibrous tissue, but of muscle tissue. They are white, dense, encapsulated masses. Fibroid tumors can be so small that they go unnoticed, or they can grow to enormous sizes. Tumors weighing over 100 pounds have been recorded. Although it is possible to develop only one fibroid tumor, most women who develop them have multiple myomas.

As many as one in three women have fibroid tumors. Happily, most are symptom free. Commonly, fibroid tumors develop toward the end of the reproductive years. Because they can result in infertility, their development can be a problem for women in their late thirties or forties who wish to have children.

Myomas that grow rapidly are more likely to be cancerous, but even then, the chances are relatively small. Fibroid tumors grow in spurts and do not develop when estrogen levels are low, a condition that occurs before the start of a woman's first period or after menopause, if she is not taking hormone replacement therapy. The biggest problem with fibroid tumors is that they can grow to a tremendous size and crowd out other organs.

Causes of Fibroid Tumors of the Uterus

It is clear that estrogen is involved to some extent in the development of fibroid tumors. When estrogen levels are at a peak, such as during pregnancy or when a woman is taking birth control pills, fibroid tumors tend to flourish. If you are near or going through menopause and you do not plan to take estrogen, any fibroid tumors you have will probably decrease or go away. The growth of fibroid tumors is probably also related to other hormones, such as growth hormone and progesterone.

Types of Fibroid Tumors

There are three types of fibroid tumors, corresponding to their location in the uterine wall. Of the three, the submucous fibroid is the most dangerous because it can cause uncontrollable bleeding. Here are details on the three types of fibroid tumors:

Intramural or interstitial tumors. This type of fibroid is located in the middle of the muscular wall of the uterus. It tends not to cause problems unless it grows to a huge size.

Subserous or subperitoneal fibroid tumors. This type of myoma grows on the outside of the uterus. It develops underneath the outer lining and can grow to a large size. This type of fibroid can become *pedunculated*, which means that it grows a stalk attached to the uterine wall. Trouble can occur if it twists on its stalk, causing extreme pain. These tumors tend not to cause problems unless they grow to a huge size.

Submucous fibroid. This type of fibroid grows on the inside of the uterus in the uterine wall under the endometrium. It can distort the shape of the uterus, causing severe bleeding. Submucous fibroid tumors can also become pedunculated.

Risk

These are the major risk factors for developing fibroid tumors:

72

Number of children. The more children you have had, the less likely that you will have fibroid tumors.

Family history. Fibroid tumors run in families.

Obesity. Because fat stores estrogen and estrogen appears to stimulate the growth of fibroid tumors, obesity is an indicator of high risk for fibroid tumors. If you are at high risk for fibroid tissues because of a family history, it is to your benefit to keep your weight down.

Race. Black women are five times more likely to develop fibroid tumors than white women.

Symptoms

The symptoms for fibroid tumors of the uterus include:

Heavy bleeding. The majority of women with symptoms experience heavy bleeding during and between periods.

Miscarriage and infertility. A big danger for many women is that fibroid tumors can result in infertility or miscarriage. The chances are probably better if fibroid tumors are removed before they get too large.

Pelvic pressure. A bloated, full, or heavy feeling may result from large fibroid tumors. The abdomen may bulge. Clothes may be tight.

Discomfort during sexual intercourse. Fibroid tumors can make normal sexual relations difficult.

Urinary, bowel, and rectal symptoms. Because fibroid tumors can crowd out nearby organs, women with myomas may have symptoms relating to problems with these organs, such as needing to urinate too frequently or difficulty with bowel movements.

Diagnosis

Most fibroid tumors are discovered by a doctor during the patient's annual physical. The area is then viewed through sonography, which uses sound waves to create a picture, to determine the number, size, and location of the tumors. Laparoscopy, viewing the abdomen with a lighted instrument, and hysterosalpingograms, using a dye and X-ray, are also sometimes used. The doctor may perform a D and C.

Myomas can feel like ovarian tumors. If there is even a slight chance that what appears to be a fibroid could be an ovarian tumor, your doctor will want to perform a laparoscopy for diagnostic purposes.

Treatment

Many gynecologists go by the rule that tumors that are larger than the size of a three-month pregnancy require a hysterectomy. However, if you have large fibroid tumors and are not uncomfortable, then there is no real reason to have your uterus removed.

Myomectomy. The procedure to surgically remove fibroid tumors from the uterus is called a myomectomy. It is a major surgical procedure. The surgery prevents the need for a hysterectomy and enables the patient to keep her uterus. After the fibroid tumors are removed, the uterus is reconstructed. Myomectomy usually results in alleviation or disappearance of heavy bleeding. A possible complication from the procedure is that scar tissue may cause some difficulties for women who wish to get pregnant. It can also weaken the uterus significantly.

A major drawback to myomectomies is that the fibroid tumors can reoccur. As long as you have a uterus, you can develop fibroid tumors.

Warning. Myomectomies are relatively new in this country, although they have been performed for many years in Europe. Many doctors do not like to perform them or are not familiar with the procedure, and therefore may suggest that the patients have hysterectomies to remove the fibroid tumors. *Be sure to get a second opinion* if you have any reason to believe this is the case with your physician.

Sometimes, during a myomectomy, surgeons switch and perform a hysterectomy because of legitimate complications such as uncontrollable heavy bleeding. However, at other times, surgeons may switch because performing a hysterectomy is easier. If you do not want your uterus, ovaries, or fallopian tubes removed, *be sure your doctor knows this*. Also *do not* sign a form giving permission for a hysterectomy to be performed if complications occur during surgery. Otherwise, you may wake up without a uterus or ovaries. When the hospital gives you a consent form to sign, write in the following:

I DO NOT GIVE PERMISSION FOR A HYSTERECTOMY TO BE PERFORMED. MY UTERUS, FALLOPIAN TUBES, AND OVARIES ARE TO REMAIN INTACT. I GIVE PERMISSION FOR A MYOMECTOMY ONLY.

A good rule of thumb when planning surgery for fibroid tumors is to locate a surgeon that has performed a large number of successful myomectomies. And make sure that the surgeon has only rarely switched to a hysterectomy during the course of a myomectomy.

Other types of surgery for fibroid tumors are less common. Myomectomies and similar procedures are sometimes performed on submucous fibroid tumors through the vagina rather than the abdomen. Some small subserous tumors can be removed with laparoscopy.

Sometimes drugs are used to treat fibroid tumors. GnRH analogs are used to create an artificial menopause and shrink tumors. However, shrinking fibroid tumors before surgery is not always a good idea. The surgeon may miss them or have trouble detecting their boundaries. Also, the drugs can bring on all the unpleasant symptoms of menopause, such as hot flashes and genital atrophy. In addition, GnRH analogs are not yet approved by the Food and Drug Administration for use with fibroid tumors.

A drug called Danocrine and progestagens are also sometimes used. However, Danocrine can cause development of masculine characteristics. Progestagens help to alleviate bleeding problems.

Hysterectomy. Fibroid tumors are the most common reason hysterectomies are performed in this country. However, in many cases, a hysterectomy can be avoided. A rule of thumb used by many gynecologists is that if the uterus is larger than a three-month pregnancy, a hysterectomy can be considered, but not before. (For more information on hysterectomies see Key 35.)

Cancerous Fibroid Tumors

Called myosarcomas or leiomyosarcomas, cancerous fibroid tumors are extremely rare. Estimates are that women have about a 1 in 200 chance that a fibroid tumor is cancerous. In the early stages, cancerous myomas can be removed with myomectomies. Often, however, the woman with cancerous fibroid tumors has to have the entire reproductive system removed.

26

OTHER CAUSES OF UTERINE BLEEDING

As discussed in Key 8, bleeding usually becomes irregular as the reproductive years begin to wane. In most cases these changes are perfectly normal. However, sometimes abnormal bleeding can occur. A number of causes of abnormal bleeding, such as fibroid tumors and different forms of cancer, are covered in other keys. This key covers common causes of abnormal bleeding not discussed elsewhere. They include adenomyosis, atrophic vaginitis, polyps, dysfunctional uterine bleeding (DUB), and endometriosis.

Adenomyosis

This is a condition that hits mostly women in their 40s and 50s who have had children. It occurs when pieces of the uterine lining break away and attach to the wall of the uterus. Each month the transplanted tissue responds to the menstrual cycle, as it would if it were still on the uterine wall. This causes enlargement and tenderness of the uterus; heavy, long periods; and cramps. It often goes away if estrogen levels drop.

Atrophic Vaginitis

As estrogen levels drop, the walls of the vagina thin out, become dry, and can become infected. Such atrophy may cause bleeding, particularly after intercourse. Estrogen or other creams can help the problem (see Key 10).

Cervical or Uterine Polyps

These are growths that develop on the uterine lining or cervical canal. They often have stems and can be removed in the doctor's office with forceps or through a D and C. Removal of polyps without stems is more complicated.

Dysfunctional Uterine Bleeding (DUB)

Doctors refer to abnormal vaginal bleeding that is not caused by tumors, inflammation, or pregnancy as dysfunctional uterine bleeding (DUB). DUB occurs most often in women over 45. One of its major causes is a change in the ovulation patterns as the reproductive system begins to wind down. During the later years of the reproductive cycle, many women do not ovulate regularly. When an egg is not released, progesterone is not produced, causing irregularity in the buildup of the uterine lining. This may result in heavy bleeding between or during periods as bits of uneven tissue break off from the lining. Other causes of DUB include the use of unopposed estrogen (estrogen without progesterone) and polycystic ovaries. Progesterone or oral contraceptives are sometimes given to restore a balance to the uterine lining.

Endometriosis

This condition occurs when pieces of the uterine lining break away, leave the uterus, and attach themselves to other organs or areas such as the ovaries, fallopian tubes, bladder, or rectum. Sometimes, endometrial tissue is even found in the lungs or nose. As with adenomyosis, each month the transplanted tissue responds to the menstrual cycle, causing swelling, pain, and bleeding. Endometriosis often results in infertility.

Diagnosis of endometriosis is usually made with laparoscopy. Treatment is controversial. Options include hormone therapy (including Danazol, which causes masculine characteristics such as facial hair), surgical removal of the implanted tissue, and, sometimes, hysterectomy.

27

FIBROCYSTIC CHANGES AND OTHER BENIGN BREAST CONDITIONS

Most women who find lumps in their breasts react with fearful images of mastectomies and breast reconstruction. But, in most cases, such lumps are *noncancerous* fibrocystic changes that have occurred in breast tissue. According to the American Cancer Society, "Fibrocystic changes are the most common cause of breast lumps in women ages 30 to 50."[1] Such changes may be referred to as fibrocystic disease, cystic disease, chronic cystic mastitis, or mammary dysplasia. However, the word *disease* is a misnomer, for fibrocystic breasts are not a disease at all, but a benign condition. In fact, if you have fibrocystic breasts, you *do not* have a higher risk of cancer, as many women fear.

About half of all women have fibrocystic breasts during their reproductive years. The condition tends to grow worse as women near the age of menopause, and the condition remains for those who take estrogen. The lumps are caused by monthly changes in the amount of and the balance between the hormones estrogen and progesterone. In response to these hormones, the breast tissue increases in firmness and cysts form in milk ducts. The cysts are fluid-filled sacs that are movable. The lumpiness is usually evident prior to menstruation when breast tissues swell.

What do fibrocystic lumps feel like? They may feel like small beads or an irregularly-shaped thickening with a lumpy or ridgelike surface. You may feel a dull ache, a feeling of

---

[1]American Cancer Society, "Fibrocystic Lumps: A Non-Disease."

heaviness, or a burning sensation, or be very tender in the area around the lump. Usually lumps are found in both breasts in the upper outer quadrant or on the underside.

Doctors usually suggest taking a mild analgesic, such as aspirin or ibuprofen, to relieve the pain and tenderness of fibrocystic breasts. Eliminating salt from the diet may help swelling. Your doctor may also suggest taking an occasional diuretic. Many women wear a larger-size bra prior to their periods. Doctors advise patients with fibrocystic breasts to avoid foods with caffeine.

Fibrocystic lumps can be aspirated in the doctor's office. Women with numerous lumps may find that they have to have a number of biopsies. Vitamin E, Danocrine, and/or Tamoxifen are sometimes prescribed. The latter two, however, cause side effects.

Fibrocystic change is the most common cause of breast lumps. However, other conditions can also cause benign lumps:

Breast cysts. Women sometimes develop cysts in their breasts that are not caused by fibrocystic changes and are not cancerous. Usually they seem to arrive suddenly and are firm, round lumps with smooth surfaces. They can be aspirated with a needle and should be biopsied.

Fat necrosis. This is another condition that can be mistaken for cancer in which calcium deposits replace dead fat cells in the breasts. Fat necrosis may occur after weight loss or with aging. Doctors usually biopsy a sample of the tissue to make sure that the calcium deposits are not the type that accompany cancer.

Fibroadenomas. These are another type of benign breast lump. Fibroadenomas usually appear by themselves and are painless. They are firm, round, and move freely when touched. Most doctors recommend removing these lumps because it is hard to distinguish them from a breast tumor called cystosarcoma, which can be cancerous.

Fibrosis. This is a benign condition in which fibrous tissue forms firm, thickened areas in the breast. Doctors usually biopsy a sample of the tissue to confirm a diagnosis.

Nipple papillomas. These are growths that appear near the nipple. They produce a bloody discharge, which should be checked by a doctor and biopsied.

Nipple polyps. These are small harmless growths that have stalks and heads. Often they are removed for cosmetic reasons.

Sclerosing adenosis. This is a benign condition in which glandular tissue replaces some of the normal tissue in the breast. The growth can be spread throughout the breast or feel like a cancerlike mass. Doctors usually biopsy a sample of the tissue to confirm a diagnosis.

28

FACTS ON CANCER AND MIDLIFE

This Key covers some basic facts on cancer and midlife. Keys 29 through 34 cover the types of reproductive system cancer that you should watch out for when you reach the age of menopause and beyond.

What Is Cancer?

Cancer is a deadly disease in which normal cells multiply uncontrollably. Eventually these cells take over healthy tissues, destroying them in the process. The cancer can spread to local sites (called *invasion*) or distant sites (called *metastasis*) in the body.

What Causes Cancer?

There are over 11 types of cancer. While most of us think of cancer as a modern disease, evidence of it has been found in dinosaur fossils. Our understanding of the causes of cancer is still limited, although some advances have been made in recent years. For example, it is known that some cancers are inherited, that lifestyle habits play a role, and that sun can cause skin melanomas. Lifestyle habits under personal control account for the majority of cancer risk. In fact, according to the American Institute for Cancer Research, eating and smoking account for more causes of cancer than all the other factors combined. Some researchers believe that cancer is caused by a virus. Others attribute cancer to personality. A number of studies have found that certain personality types develop cancer more often than others. For example, one study found that women who do not cope well with stress and suppress anger and other deep emotions are particularly susceptible to cancer of the breast.

How Does Cancer Develop?

Cancer can hit at any age, but the incidence and risk rise significantly with age. Most cases strike in midlife and beyond. Cancer develops in response to a carcinogen, which may be introduced into the body by a number of different everyday activities such as eating, drinking, or breathing. Under normal circumstances the body deactivates the carcinogen and filters it out of the system. But sometimes the carcinogen may bind to the DNA of a cell, where it is passed on to the next generation of cells. Any cell in the body can become cancerous, and if the cancer spreads, the cancerous cells will resemble the original.

It may take years before a tumor develops and is noticed by the individual or picked up by medical tests. In fact, it is possible to develop cancer twenty or thirty years after being exposed to a carcinogen. This is one of the reasons most cases of cancer emerge during midlife or later.

It is thought that some agents can inhibit or promote cancer. For example, some vitamins or minerals may inhibit cancer, while dietary fat, smoking, certain foods (salt-cured, smoked, and charcoal-broiled), and too much sun exposure have been recognized as promoters of cancer.

Cancer Facts

1. In 1992 about 1,130,000 people will be diagnosed with cancer and about 520,000 will die of the disease. Approximately 1,400 people in the United States die of cancer each day.[1]
2. One in five deaths in this country is from cancer. In 1991 an estimated 514,000 Americans died of cancer. According to the American Cancer Society, if present trends continue, 76 million Americans now living will eventually develop the disease. This means that cancer eventually strikes three in four families.

---

[1] Unless otherwise noted, the statistics and recommendations in this section are from *Cancer Facts and Figures* (American Cancer Society, 1992).

3. The good news is that today there are 4 million survivors of cancer who were diagnosed over five years ago. (Most of these can be considered cured, which means that they now have no evidence of the disease and have the same life expectancy that they would have without cancer.) Of those people diagnosed with cancer, about 50 percent live at least five years.
4. Women fare better than men when it comes to cancer. Cancer deaths for women have dropped 5 percent over the past 30 years, while the rate for men has gone up 16 percent.[2] The improvement for women is primarily due to a drop in uterine, stomach, and bladder cancer. For women, the most prevalent cancers are breast, colon, rectum, lung, and uterus.

Protecting Yourself

Regular self-examination and screening can detect two forms of cancer that can strike women in midlife—breast and cervical cancer. Early screening allows physicians to more precisely stage cancer growth and provide effective treatment. (For more information on screening for breast and cervical cancer see Keys 29 and 30.)

Cancer Treatment

Cancer is treated through surgery, radiation, radioactive substances, chemotherapy, hormones, and immunotherapy. Advances are being made in treating the many different types of cancer. For example, research has revealed the importance of oncogenes. Found in tumors, oncogenes are involved in the change of normal cells to cancer cells. Their detection will eventually enable doctors to learn which tumors may reoccur after surgery and to identify family members at risk for certain types of cancer. Another important finding is growth factor, which stimulates normal bone marrow cells to withstand

---

[2]*Prevention's Giant Book of Health Facts* (Emmaus, PA: Rodale Press, 1991), p. 115.

very high doses of drugs used to treat cancer. A particularly fascinating treatment currently being worked on is a microscopic submarine fueled by glucose which would go on a search-and-destroy mission through the bloodstream looking for cancer. If it finds any, it would escort it to the kidneys and out the system through urination.

Cancer Prevention

Because the risk of developing cancer increases with each additional year of life, it is particularly important to work at preventing cancer during midlife. Here is a summary of the American Cancer Society's recommendations for factors to avoid that can lead to the development of cancer.

Smoking. Cigarette smoking is responsible for 79 percent of lung cancer cases among women. Smoking accounts for about 30 percent of all cancer deaths. Those who smoke two or more packs of cigarettes a day have lung cancer mortality rates 15 to 25 times greater than nonsmokers.

Sunlight. Almost all of the more than 600,000 cases of skin cancer diagnosed each year in the United States are sun-related.

Ionizing radiation. Excessive exposure to ionizing radiation can increase cancer risk. (Most medical and dental X rays are adjusted to deliver the lowest dose possible.) Excessive radon exposure in homes may increase risk of lung cancer, especially in cigarette smokers.

Nutrition and diet. Risk of colon, breast, and uterine cancers increases in obese people. High-fat diets may contribute to the development of cancers of the breast, colon, and prostate. High-fiber foods might help reduce risk of colon cancer. A varied diet containing plenty of vegetables and fruits rich in vitamins A and C may reduce risk for a wide range of cancers. Salt-cured, smoked, and nitrite-cured foods have been linked to esophagus and stomach cancer.

Alcohol. Oral cancer and cancers of the larynx, throat, esophagus, and liver occur more frequently among heavy drinkers of alcohol especially when accompanied by cigarette smoking or tobacco chewing.

Smokeless tobacco. Use of chewing tobacco or snuff increases the risk of cancer of the mouth, larynx, throat, and esophagus and is a highly addictive habit.

Estrogen. Estrogen treatment to control menopausal symptoms increases risk of endometrial cancer. However, including progesterone in estrogen replacement therapy helps to minimize the risk. Consultation with a physician will help assess personal risks and benefits.

Occupational hazards. Exposure to several different industrial agents (nickel, chromate, asbestos, vinyl chloride, and so on) increases risk of various cancers. Risk from asbestos is greatly increased when combined with cigarette smoking.

When to See a Doctor

The American Cancer Society recommends that you see a doctor right away if you have any of the following symptoms:
- A sore that doesn't get better
- A nagging cough or an unusually hoarse voice
- Indigestion (very bad upset stomach more than once in a while)
- Problems with swallowing
- Changes in a wart or mole
- Unusual bleeding or discharge
- Thick spot or lump in breast or elsewhere
- Change in bowel or bladder habits

29

BREAST CANCER

Breast cancer is the most common form of cancer among women. It accounts for one in three cancers that strike women. Women over 50 develop about three-fourths of all breast cancers. In 1992 175,000 women were expected to develop breast cancer.

There are two important facts to remember about this disease. First, if you have close relatives, particularly a mother or sister, who have had the disease, you are at *very high risk* for developing it yourself.

The second fact may be a surprise: While women who have breast cancer in their family histories are at very high risk, the vast majority of women who develop the disease do *not* have relatives with breast cancer. In other words, not having a family history of the disease is no guarantee that you won't develop cancerous breast tumors. In fact, nearly 80 percent of women with breast cancer have *no risk factors* whatsoever, including no family history of the disease! These facts are particularly important in view of the fact that today all women have a *1 in 9 chance* of developing breast cancer, compared to 1 in 14 in 1960.[1]

Causes of Breast Cancer

A great deal of attention has been paid recently to fat in the diet as a major culprit behind breast cancer. For example, researchers have found that, in countries where the diet is low in fat, breast cancer rates are also low. But when immigrant groups, such as the Japanese, move to countries such as ours where fat is a large part of the diet, their rates of breast cancer go up.

---

[1]These statistics are from the American Cancer Society and are controversial because of the method used for tabulation.

Risk Factors for Breast Cancer

As mentioned, it is important to remember that nearly 80 percent of women with breast cancer have *no* risk factors! This startling fact points out the need to be diligent in monitoring your body for any suspicious changes that could be indicative of a cancerous growth. Breast cancer develops over a number of years. It can be growing long before any symptoms appear.

Important risk factors for breast cancer are:

Age. As mentioned above, women over 50 account for about three-fourths of all breast cancers. The average age of women diagnosed with breast cancer is 62.

Race. White people are at greater risk than blacks.

Late menopause.

Delayed childbearing. Women who had their first child at age 18 have about one-third the risk of women who first gave birth after 30 or have no children.

Early menses.

Obesity.

Family history. Fifteen to twenty percent of breast cancers are familial. The risk increases greatly if more than one breast of a close family member has been cancerous. In breast cancer that is inherited, the average age of diagnosis is 44.

Dense breast tissue. Women whose breasts are composed of dense tissue are at higher risk than those whose breasts are mostly fatty tissue.

High-fat diet. There is a five to ten times difference in deaths due to breast cancer between countries with traditionally low-fat diets and those with high-fat diets.

Birth control pills. Some studies have shown that using birth control pills is associated with an increased risk of breast cancer while others have shown a decrease.

The younger you were when you had your first child and the more children you have had, the better your chances for not developing breast tumors. Breast-feeding also decreases your chances.

Fibrocystic Breasts

Women with fibrocystic breasts (see Key 27) may have a difficult time performing a monthly breast self-exam (BSE). It is far too easy to miss a cancerous lump. If you have fibrocystic breasts, it is important to get special instruction on how to perform breast exams from your doctor or your closest American Cancer Society chapter.

Estrogen and Breast Cancer

Many women are concerned about whether estrogen is linked to breast cancer. Numerous studies have shown that there is *no connection* between breast cancer and estrogen replacement therapy. Some studies have shown that HRT can actually help prevent it. For example, a study of more than 5,500 women conducted by Dr. R. Don Gambell, Jr. in Georgia found that women on estrogen or estrogen/progesterone had a *lower* incidence of breast cancer than women who took no hormones at all. However, if you have breast cancer it is important to know whether it is *estrogen dependent*. If so, you should never take estrogen. In such cases, estrogen is not responsible for causing the tumor, but can make it grow faster. On the other hand, if you have a breast cancer that is not estrogen dependent, taking estrogen could shrink it.

Symptoms

Breast cancer can have many symptoms. It is important to get to know your breasts well so that you will know what is normal and what is not. Early detection is very important, because the sooner breast tumors are found and treated, the better the chances for recovery. *When breast cancer is detected before it has spread, the survival rate is 90 percent or more.* But, if the cancer has had time to spread, the chances drop to 60 percent.

Here are some warning signs for breast cancer from the National Cancer Institute:
• A lump or thickening in the breast or under the arm
• A change in the size or shape of the breast

- Discharge from the nipple
- A change in the color or feel of the skin of the breast or ring around the nipple (the areola), such as dimpling, puckering, or scaliness)

And the American Cancer Society (ACS) adds:

- soreness of the skin.
- a nipple that becomes drawn into the chest, changes shape, or becomes crusty.
- any pain or tenderness that lasts through the menstrual cycle.

Screening for Cancer

Here are the American Cancer Society guidelines for screening breasts for cancer:

1. Women 20 years of age and older should perform breast self-examination every month.
2. Women 20 to 40 should have a physical examination of the breasts every three years, and women over 40 should have a physical examination of the breasts every year.
3. Women between the ages of 35 and 39 should have a baseline mammogram.
4. Women age 40 to 49 should have a physical examination of the breast annually, and mammography should be performed at intervals of one to two years.
5. Women 50 years of age and older should have a mammogram every year when feasible. (The National Cancer Institute suggests that this should be *every year after age 40.*)

Mammography

X-ray examination of the breast (mammography) is particularly important in detecting breast cancers that are too small to be picked up by breast self-examination or by a physician. In fact, when women have breast tumors that are found in the early stage, the chance of survival is 100 percent. In several studies, a reduction of 30 percent or more in deaths due to breast cancer were found in women over 50 who received mammography screening. Another study found that women in their 40s who have annual mammographies can reduce their risk of dying of breast disease by 26 percent.

Mammography machines now use very low doses of radiation. No one should worry that the radiation used in mammography will induce cancer. It is important, however, to make sure that the machine used for your test gives a *two-view exam* using no more than 1 rad of radiation or less, as recommended by the American Cancer Society. Mammography may cause temporary pain, particularly for women with large breasts.

Medicare will now cover screening mammograms, and in a small number of states, Medicaid will cover them.

Diagnosis

The American Cancer Society (ACS) stresses that mammography does not pick up all cancers. In fact, doctors estimate that the test has a 15 to 20 percent failure rate. ACS recommends the following three tests for detection of breast cancer in women without symptoms: breast self-examination (BSE), breast exams by a physician or other health professional, and mammography. Seventy-five percent of all breast cancers are found by women themselves. When women have suspicious lumps, all areas of the breast should be examined with mammography and a biopsy is the only way to determine if cancer is present.

To diagnose breast cancer, your doctor will perform a careful physical exam and ask you about your family medical history. The doctor will probably do one of the following tests:

Palpation. The doctor will carefully feel the breast to examine the lump—its size, texture, and motility.

Aspiration. The doctor may use a thin needle to remove fluid or a small amount of tissue from a breast lump. This may show whether the lump is a fluid-filled cyst, which is not cancer, or a solid mass, which may or may not be cancer.

Mammography. X-rays of the breast will give the doctor important information about breast lumps. Mammograms can also show tumors that are too small to be felt.

Imaging techniques. Sometimes doctors order imaging tests along with mammography. *Ultrasound* is a test that sends high-frequency sound waves, which cannot be heard by humans, into the breast. The pattern of echoes is shown on a monitor. This test is sometimes referred to as a sonagram. *Thermography* is a test that measures and records heat patterns in the breast. *Diaphanography* is a test that is done by shining a bright light through the breast.

Biopsy. A biopsy is the only sure way to know that cancer is present. It is a surgical procedure that takes out part or all of a lump or suspicious area. The tissue is studied under a microscope by a pathologist.

Hormone receptor tests. If the biopsy shows that cancer is present, laboratory tests called *estrogen* and *progesterone receptor* tests are usually performed on the cancer cells. These tests can determine if hormones promote the growth of the cancer, and will help determine whether hormone treatment will be useful.

If the lump is cancerous, the doctor will order other tests to determine the nature of the cancer and whether or not it has spread. These tests will also help determine the *stage* of the cancer.

Doctors use this staging system for breast cancer:
1. *Carcinoma in situ* is very early breast cancer. Cancer is found in a local area and in only a few layers of cells.
2. *Stage I* means the tumor is no larger than 2 centimeters (cm), about an inch, and has not spread beyond the breast.
3. *Stage II* means the tumor is from 2 cm to 5 cm, about 1 to 2 inches, and/or has spread to the *lymph nodes* under the arm.
4. *Stage III* means the cancer is larger than 5 cm, about 2 inches. It has spread to other tissues near the breast.
5. *Stage IV* means the cancer has spread to other organs of the body, most often the bones, liver, lungs, or brain.

Treatment of Breast Cancer

A decade ago breast cancer was synonymous with removal

of the entire breast, the chest muscles under the breast, and the underarm chest muscles (a radical mastectomy). Happily, this procedure is rarely done today. Since the early 1980s there has been tremendous progress in the early identification and treatment of breast cancer. And new developments are occurring all the time. For example, lumpectomy removes the breast lump only, and a partial mastectomy removes the lump and a wedge of normal tissue surrounding it. Both are followed by radiation therapy.

Breast Self-Examination (BSE)

It is important to do a BSE once a month. Key 30 offers a demonstration of one method of performing BSE. As mentioned previously, if you have fibrocystic breasts, you should get special instruction from a health professional. It is extremely important that BSE be as thorough as possible.

BSE should be performed at the same time each month so that you can become familiar with how your breasts feel at that particular time. If you still have periods, you should perform your exam two or three days after your period ends when your breast are less full.

30

HOW TO PERFORM BREAST SELF-EXAMINATION

It is important to perform a breast self-examination (BSE) every month, either two or three days after your period (if you still have one), or at the same time each month. The more often you practice BSE, the more familiar with your breast you will become and the easier it will be to detect suspicious changes. Getting in the habit of performing regular breast self-examinations can save your life.

Here is a demonstration of one method from the American Institute for Cancer Research:

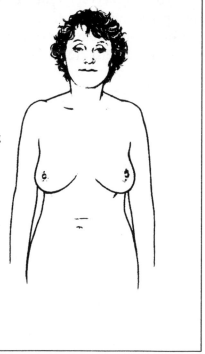

1 Stand before a mirror. Check both breasts for anything unusual. Look for a discharge from the nipples, puckering, dimpling, or scaling of the skin.

The next two steps are done to check for any change in the shape or contour of your breasts. As you do them, you should be able to feel your chest muscles tighten.

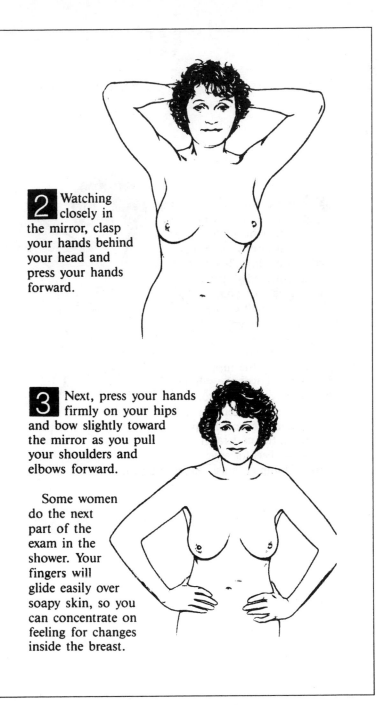

2 Watching closely in the mirror, clasp your hands behind your head and press your hands forward.

3 Next, press your hands firmly on your hips and bow slightly toward the mirror as you pull your shoulders and elbows forward.

Some women do the next part of the exam in the shower. Your fingers will glide easily over soapy skin, so you can concentrate on feeling for changes inside the breast.

4 Raise your left arm. Use three or four fingers of your right hand to feel your left breast firmly, carefully, and thoroughly. Beginning at the outer edge, press the flat part of your fingers in small circles, moving the circles slowly around the breast. Gradually work toward the nipple. Be sure to cover the whole breast. Pay special attention to the area between the breast and the underarm, including the underarm area itself. Feel for any unusual lump or mass under the skin.

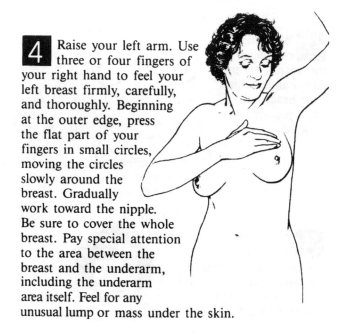

5 Gently squeeze the nipple and look for a discharge. (If you have any discharge during the month—whether or not it is during BSE—see your doctor.) Repeat the exam on your right breast.

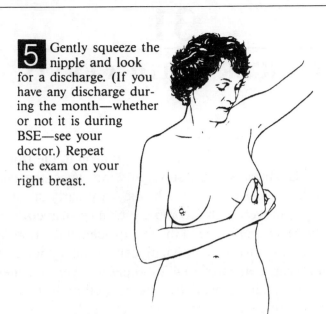

6 Steps 4 and 5 should be repeated lying down. Lie flat on your back, with your left arm over your head and a pillow or folded towel under your left shoulder. This position flattens the breast and makes it easier to check it. Use the same circular motion described above. Repeat on your right breast.

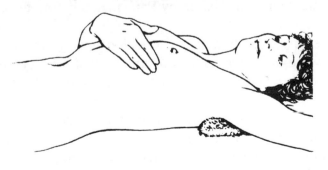

The preceding material is reprinted with permission from the American Institute for Cancer Research.

31

CANCER OF THE CERVIX

Cervical cancer is a common cancer of the female reproductive system. However, there is no reason to die from the disease today, because it is a slow-growing cancer that can be detected in the doctor's office in the very early stages and surgically removed with a complete chance of recovery. In fact, cervical cancer is one of the few cancers with a *decreasing* death rate. Invasive cervical cancer now hits 13,000 women a year, compared to 47,000 cases a year for uterine cancer. The major reason for the reduction is that more women now understand the need to get regular pelvic exams and Pap smears.

Causes of Cervical Cancer
While the cause of cervical cancer is not certain, it is clear that the disease starts as an inflammatory reaction that develops into abnormal cells over time. Cervical cancer takes several years to develop, and its forerunner of abnormal cells (dysplasia) can be picked up by Pap smears before the cells develop into cancer.

There is speculation that cervical cancer is caused by extensive sexual intercourse. It is known that it occurs more frequently in women who experienced early sexual activity, multiple partners, and early childbirth. One possibility is that semen causes inflammation. Another is that cervical cancer is related to sexually transmitted diseases such as the human papilloma virus (HPV). A reoccurring inflammation or infection of the cervix (cervicitis) might also contribute to the disease. Women who are at particularly high risk should have Pap smears twice a year.

Risk Factors for Cervical Cancer

Cervical cancer could be eliminated as a cause of death if all women had annual *Pap tests*. Unfortunately, less than 40 percent of women do so. Cervical cancer can occur at any age but is more likely to hit in midlife. This type of cancer is most common among women whose sexual experiences began early in life, with multiple sexual partners, and with early childbearing. Recently the human papilloma virus (HPV) has been implicated as causes of cervical cancer.

Here is a summary of important risk factors for cervical cancer:

Age. Cervical cancer is more likely to occur between the ages of 40 and 55.

Race. If you are black or Puerto Rican, your risk is higher than if you are a member of other ethnic groups.

Socioeconomic level. Women with lower socioeconomic levels are at higher risk.

Early childbearing.

Early sexual experiences.

Multiple sexual partners.

Human papilloma virus (HPV).

Cervicitis. Inflammation of the cervix.

Symptoms

There are no symptoms for early cervical cancer. It can only be detected by a Pap smear. In more advanced stages, pain may be felt and irregular bleeding may occur. Other symptoms that should be checked promptly are unusual vaginal discharge, problems urinating, and severe constipation.

Diagnosis

Cervical cancer is first picked up by Pap smears and then diagnosed by colposcopy or biopsy of the cervix. If it is picked up in the precancerous or early stages, the growth can be surgically removed. In such cases the patient has a 100 percent chance of survival. Deaths from cervical cancer usually occur because the *diagnosis was made too late* in the disease process.

Here are details on the diagnostic tests used for cervical cancer:

Pap tests. The Pap test is used for analyzing the cells of the vagina, endocervix, and cervix. The doctor uses a speculum to take samples from the cervix, which are analyzed by a laboratory. The Pap test can detect 90 percent of early cancerous growths. According to the *Merck Manual,* its use has reduced deaths from cervical cancer by over 50 percent.

The Pap test is usually conducted in the doctor's office during routine annual physicals. However, as mentioned earlier, women who are at high risk for cervical cancer should have Pap smears more often.

D and C (dilatation and curettage). A D and C may be part of the diagnostic process for cervical cancer. Doctors sometimes perform D and Cs in hospitals, using general anesthesia.

Vabra aspiration. This procedure may be used for diagnosis. It involves removing the endometrium by using low-pressure suction.

Colposcopy. A lighted magnifying instrument is used to examine the vaginal walls and cervix and identify the specific areas where the cancer is located. Colposcopy is used to pinpoint areas for biopsy.

Cervical biopsy. This procedure involves removing a sample of abnormal tissue from the cervix for examination under a microscope.

Conization or cone biopsy. This procedure, in which a cone-shaped piece of the cervix is removed, may be used for diagnosis or treatment. A cone biopsy is a major surgical procedure performed in a hospital with a scalpel or laser.

Schiller's test. This test is used to pinpoint areas for biopsy when colposcopy is not available. An iodine solution is applied to the cervix. Abnormal areas will not absorb the stain, while normal tissue will turn a dark brown.

In addition, your doctor will have other tests performed to see if the cancer has spread.

Treatment of Cervical Cancer

Cervical cancer can be removed with a cone biopsy if it is *in situ* —in other words, in the early stages, contained in one area, with the cells occurring in a few layers. Many women who now have cone biopsies, would in previous years have had hysterectomies. Doctors usually require Pap smears every three months after a cone biopsy to make sure that all of the cancer has been removed and that it does not recur. *Laser ablation cones* are sometimes performed in place of cone biopsies. In this procedure, the tissue surrounding the abnormal cells is vaporized instead of being removed. Alternative treatments are *cryosurgery*, in which the abnormal cells are destroyed by freezing, and *cauterization*, in which the tissue is burned. Some doctors advise removing the uterus to prevent spreading of the cancer.

Invasive cancer, in which the diseased tissue has spread, is treated with extensive hysterectomy (see Key 35), irradiation, and cobalt therapy. Tumors reoccur or persist about 35 percent of the time. Radiation treatment for early invasive cancer has about a 60 to 90 percent success rate.

32

CANCER OF THE UTERUS (CANCER OF THE ENDOMETRIUM)

Uterine cancer is cancer of the lining of the uterus. (It is also referred to as cancer of the endometrium.) Each year 47,000 women are diagnosed with invasive cancer of the uterus. However, uterine cancer is far less deadly than cancer of the cervix. It is also most commonly thought of in relation to hormone replacement therapy.[1]

Estrogen and Uterine Cancer

During the early 1970s, uterine cancer increased, because of the number of women taking estrogen without the protection of combining it with progesterone. However, as mentioned previously, most experts believe that an increase in uterine cancer is no longer a danger when estrogen is used in conjunction with progesterone.

Other Causes of Uterine Cancer

A diet high in fat has been linked to uterine cancer. Also, a condition called *adenomatous hyperplasia*, which is an overgrowth of endometrial tissue, can develop into uterine cancer. The condition is thought to occur with hormone imbalances in which ovulation does not take place. Adenomatous hyperplasia is usually treated by progesterone therapy or hysterectomy.

Risk Factors for Uterine Cancer

Uterine cancer occurs most often after menopause. Seventy-five percent of all cases occur after age fifty. Women who have never had children, have a delayed menopause, take estrogen

---

[1]Robert Berkow, ed., *The Merck Manual*, 15th ed. (Rahway, NJ: Merck and Co., 1987), p. 1727.

without progestin, or have a hormone imbalance of high estrogen levels with infrequent ovulation are most likely to develop this type of cancer. Other risk factors include overweight, diabetes, high blood pressure, and a family history of the disease. The danger of getting uterine cancer rises with income.

Symptoms

The major symptom of uterine cancer is abnormal bleeding. If you are no longer having menstrual periods and you have *vaginal bleeding*, see a doctor right away. A watery discharge may precede bleeding. As many as one in three cases of postmenopausal bleeding is due to uterine cancer. The symptoms for women who still have periods are increased menstrual flow and bleeding between periods.

Diagnosis

The Pap smear is not a reliable detector of uterine cancer. It picks up this type of cancer only occasionally. Your doctor may schedule a D and C, *endometrial biopsy*, or Vabra technique if cancer is suspected (see Key 31). Aspiration curettage, which is an office procedure similar to a D and C but taking a smaller amount of tissue, may also be used. However, a procedure called a fractional curettage is usually performed. This procedure provides grading of the tumor and can determine if the cancer has advanced into the cervix.

Some doctors advise endometrial biopsies, the analysis of uterine tissue, around the time of menopause. Others routinely advise that annual biopsies be taken at the same time as the annual Pap smear. Certainly, anyone in a high risk category, such as an overweight person or one with a family history of the disease should consider regular endometrial biopsies.

Treatment of Uterine Cancer

This type of cancer usually results in complete hysterectomy, chemotherapy, and radiation. Progesterone may prevent spread of the cancer. The success rate for treatment is high if the cancer is found early. The five-year survival rate is about 90 percent. Most women with this type of cancer cannot take estrogen.

33

CANCER OF THE OVARIES

Ovarian cancer is responsible for one in five cancers of the reproductive tract. While this type of cancer occurs far less often than endometrial or cervical cancer, it takes almost as many lives, because it is a fast-moving cancer and detection is difficult until it is in the advanced stages. In fact, in 70 to 80 percent of cases, the disease is extensive.[1] Each year, ovarian cancer is diagnosed in about 20,700 women, and 12,500 women die from the disease.

Causes of Ovarian Cancer

The cause of ovarian cancer is unknown. However, the more years you ovulate, the higher the risk that you will develop ovarian cancer.[2] Unlike breast and uterine cancers of the reproductive tract, there is no indication that cancer of the ovaries is in any way connected to estrogen. In fact, many physicians believe that estrogen helps protect against this type of cancer. There is speculation that leutenizing hormone (LH) and follicle-stimulating hormone (FSH) may irritate the ovaries in some way, however (see Key 3).

Risk Factors for Ovarian Cancer

Ovarian cancer occurs more often after menopause and in women who are overweight. The peak occurrences are in women in their 50s. Women who have never had children are at higher risk than those who have. Curiously, the more children you have had, the lower the risk. In addition, use of birth control pills reduces risk for the disease. Women who

---

[1] Robert Berkow, ed., *The Merck Manual*, 15th ed. (Rahway, NJ: Merck and Co., 1987), p. 1727.

[2] Sadja Greenwood, *Menopause Naturally* (Volcano, CA: Volcano Press, 1989), p. 53.

have had breast, intestinal, or rectal cancer are at increased risk. Women who have worked in the electrical, rubber, or textile industries may be at higher risk, as well as women who have had pelvic radiation. Another factor to consider is a family history of the disease. Also, the more years you ovulate, the higher the risk of ovarian cancer.[3]

Symptoms

Symptoms of ovarian cancer are often vague and difficult to detect. Abdominal swelling is the most common sign. Early symptoms include digestive problems such as gas pains, bloating, and constipation. In fact, unusual *gas pains* and *related symptoms* should always be investigated by a gynecologist. Sometimes there is a need to urinate often. In advanced stages of ovarian cancer, fatigue, pelvic pain, anemia, and emaciation may occur. Sometimes there is a buildup of fluid in the abdomen.

Diagnosis

After menopause, the ovaries of women who do not take estrogen shrink and are difficult to feel. If you are past menopause, if you are not taking estrogen, and if your ovaries can be felt during a pelvic examination, your doctor will probably suspect cancer. In premenopausal women or women on estrogen, if the ovaries feel enlarged or there is an unusual growth, cancer is suspected. Diagnostic tests may include ultrasound, X-rays, and/or a CAT scan (computerized X ray).

Treatment of Ovarian Cancer

This type of cancer usually results in removal of the ovaries and fallopian tubes. The *omentum*, a part of the abdominal lining where cancer spreads easily, is also often removed. One in four ovarian tumors removed by surgery is malignant. Surgery is usually done in combination with chemotherapy. Radiation may be used in certain circumstances. Unhappily, the cure rate for ovarian cancer is low, because it is usually so far advanced by the time it is detected.

---

[3] Greenwood, p. 53.

34

VAGINAL AND
VULVAR CANCER

While these two types of cancer are relatively uncommon, they are included here because they occur most often after menopause.

Vaginal Cancer

Vaginal cancer, fortunately, is rare. It usually develops in the outer skin area layer of the vagina and in the upper half of the vagina. Sometimes it spreads from the uterus.

Risk Factors for Vaginal Cancer. Vaginal cancer has been linked to women's exposure to a synthetic estrogen, DES (diethylstilbestrol), in the mother's uterus. It has also been found that some strains of human papilloma virus (HPV) can cause this type of cancer.

Symptoms. Vaginal bleeding is an early indication of cancer. Pain is felt in more advanced cases and urinary symptoms may occur. Pain may be felt during sexual intercourse.

Diagnosis. Vaginal cancer may be found with a Pap smear. For this reason, women who have had hysterectomies should continue to have regular Pap smears.

Treatment of Vaginal Cancer. If vaginal cancer is discovered early, it can be removed by surgery. Irradiation may be used.

Vulvar Cancer

Vulvar cancer occurs only slightly more often than vaginal cancer. It usually strikes older women.

Risk Factors for Vulvar Cancer. As with vaginal cancer, some strains of papilloma virus can cause this type of cancer.

Symptoms. Itching is the first symptom of vulvar cancer. The lesion may look like a wart. A major danger with this type of cancer is that women discount the symptoms. Doctors may even treat the itching and ignore the condition that is developing.

Diagnosis. Biopsy is used for diagnosis.

Treatment of Vulvar Cancer. After colposcopy (see Key 31), a vulvectomy is performed, a surgical procedure to remove the vulva.

35

HYSTERECTOMY

Women are often told that they need to have hysterectomies to cure problems ranging from fibroid tumors to prolapsed uteruses. However, in far too many cases, they don't really need to undergo such major surgery. About 650,000 women a year have hysterectomies, many of which are elective. In other words, unless a fatal disease is involved, the surgery is performed to increase the quality of life and is the decision of the patient. For example, women have hysterectomies to stop excessive bleeding, relieve pain, or remove harmless, but large, fibroid tumors.

The decision to have a hysterectomy should always be thought through very carefully. Any doctor who insists that you need one should be questioned. Even if you have cancer, hysterectomy is not always necessary.

Types of Hysterectomy

Hysterectomy refers to removal of the uterus only. It ends menstruation and the ability to give birth. Also, some women who have hysterectomies go through menopause earlier than they would otherwise. There are many different types of hysterectomies. It is important to know what type of operation your doctor plans to perform. Each kind of hysterectomy is done for specific reasons with different results.

Here is a summary of the different types of hysterectomy:

Total hysterectomy. This is the most common type of hysterectomy. The entire uterus is removed, including the cervix. Menstrual periods stop, but because the ovaries are not removed, the monthly hormonal changes still occur.

Supracervical, subtotal, or partial hysterectomy. The top of the uterus is taken out and the cervix remains. This is a less extensive and less dangerous operation than a total hysterectomy. It is an important alternative for women who feel that removal of the cervix might decrease the enjoyment of sexual intercourse. In addition, there is less risk that the ureter and bladder will be damaged during surgery. However, it does not eliminate the risk of cervical cancer and makes treatment for it more difficult if it occurs. Supracervical hysterectomies are becoming more common, because of increased awareness of the role that the cervix plays in sexual pleasure.

Oophorectomy. In this operation one ovary is removed.

Bilateral oophorectomy. In this procedure both ovaries are removed.

Radical hysterectomy. This operation involves removal of the uterus, the top third of the vagina, uterine ligaments, and some lymph nodes from the pelvic area. It is a higher risk operation than a subtotal hysterectomy and is reserved for cervical or endometrial cancer. Fortunately, this operation is performed less frequently now because the increased use of Pap smears permits the early detection and treatment of cancer before it spreads. If you are scheduled for a radical hysterectomy, ask your doctor about a *modified* or *type II* radical hysterectomy, which allows better chances of maintaining normal bowel and bladder function.

Hysterectomy with unilateral salpingo-oophorectomy. This mouthful means removal of the uterus, one ovary, and one fallopian tube.

Hysterectomy with bilateral salpingo-oophorectomy. This surgery involves the removal of the uterus, both ovaries, and both fallopian tubes. It is performed when invasive cancer, endometriosis, or infection has spread.

Saving Your Ovaries

Estimates are that 25 to 40 percent of hysterectomies include removal of the ovaries. Many doctors push removing perfectly healthy ovaries with a variation of this remote rationale: "Once you are in menopause they aren't doing you any good anyway, so while we have you open to take your uterus out, we might as well take your ovaries out and prevent the threat of cancer."

There are two major things wrong with this explanation. First, the ovaries continue to produce a number of hormones after menopause. Scientists aren't even sure what role some of these hormones play and what the effects are of eliminating them. In addition, they are not restored by hormone replacement therapy. Second, unless a woman is at very high risk, it does not make sense to remove perfectly healthy ovaries because of the very remote threat of cancer. As discussed in Key 33, ovarian cancer is relatively rare.

Vaginal or Abdominal Hysterectomy

Hysterectomies may be performed vaginally or through the abdomen. In vaginal surgery the uterus is removed through the vagina. Two advantages are that there is no abdominal incision and recovery is faster. One in four hysterectomies is vaginal.

Vaginal hysterectomies are performed often on older women who require surgery for prolapsed uteruses. However, there are many circumstances when this approach cannot be used, including partial hysterectomies or when the uterus is enlarged. Vaginal hysterectomies also make removal of the ovaries more difficult.

Abdominal hysterectomies are the most common. In this procedure, the doctor actually makes cuts in both the abdomen and the vagina. (The uterus is detached and then removed through the vagina.) The abdominal cut is made in a vertical or horizontal line, starting at the navel and reaching to the pubic bone. While this operation provides the surgeon with access to the organs he is working on, the rate of complications is also higher.

If you are scheduled for an abdominal hysterectomy, you may want to talk to your surgeon about having a "bikini cut," which runs along the top of the pubic hair line. However, if your surgery is being performed because of cancer, large ovarian cysts, or an enlarged uterus, your doctor will probably not want to do a "bikini cut."

According to the American College of Obstetricians and Gynecologists, the conditions that suggest hysterectomies are:

• very unusual bleeding not controlled by other treatment.

• severe endometriosis (see Key 26).

• fibroid tumors of the uterus with increasing size, pain, or bleeding (see Key 25).

• increasing pain related to the uterus and not controlled by other treatment, possibly caused by pelvic adhesions.

• defects in pelvic supports (see Key 23).

• early malignant changes or changes that may lead to cancer of the uterus.

• pregnancy-related problems.

Hysterectomy, the Down Side

Hysterectomies are major surgery, performed under general anesthesia and requiring weeks of recovery. Between one and two deaths occur for every one thousand hysterectomies.[1] And one to two in four women having hysterectomies run into complications such as fever and heavy bleeding.

There are other problems that also can occur. For example, the risk of having a pulmonary embolism is increased. In addition, the organs that are being worked on in surgery are crowded in with the bladder, rectum, and other organs, and sometimes the surgeon will accidentally cut or otherwise damage other organs.

Some women report experiencing depression after a hysterectomy. Others experience a decrease in sexual desire. In a

---

[1] "Hysterectomy and Its Alternatives," *Consumer Reports*, September 1990, p. 604.

study by the U.S. Centers for Disease Control in the early 1980s, more than half the women reported no change in sexual desire, 9 percent noticed decreased desire, and 9 percent said that they had *increased* sexual desire after their hysterectomies. Another complication that can occur is residual ovary syndrome, in which scar tissue forms around the ovaries.

Who Gets Hysterectomies?

When we look at the statistics describing who gets hysterectomies, some curious facts emerge. Only 1 in 10 hysterectomies are performed for cancer. Hysterectomy rates vary between different regions of the United States. Also, if your doctor receives a fee for the operation, you are far more likely to have a hysterectomy than if you are a member of a health plan, such as a health maintenance organization. Finally, hysterectomies are most often performed for fibroid tumors, endometriosis, and uterine prolapse, all of which could be treated with other procedures.[2]

There are specific reasons that doctors like to perform hysterectomies. Here are some:

• They're lucrative.

• Monitoring the gynecological problem that is causing the need for the operation is much more trouble than just taking everything out.

• Hysterectomies are far easier to perform than other more complicated procedures that address the same problem, such as myomectomy.

• Many doctors don't know how to do other operations such as myomectomies.

[2]Gale Maleskey and Charles Inlander, *Take This Book to the Gynecologist with You* (Reading, MA: Addison-Wesley, 1991), p. 110.

After taking all of the warnings into account, there are times when hysterectomies are appropriate—specifically, for:

- life-threatening cancer.

- severe, uncontrollable infection.

- severe, uncontrollable bleeding.

- life-threatening blockages of organs due to growths on the uterus.

If you have been told that you require a hysterectomy for one of these problems, it is important to get a second opinion. If the decision is made to go forward, locate a surgeon who performs complicated hysterectomies often, at least twice or more per week. Also be sure that you know exactly what is going to be removed and how long your recovery period will be. In addition, if your ovaries are being removed, it is important to ask your doctor about your options for hormone replacement therapy.

36

IF YOU ARE HAVING SURGERY

If your docter tells you that you need to have a hysterectomy, myomectomy, lumpectomy, or other major surgery, you should get a second opinion. And if the second opinion does not agree with the first, get a third opinion. Most health plans will cover the costs.

Most surgical procedures can be performed regardless of age. According to a recent Mayo Clinic study that looked at whether surgery was risky for people in older age groups, age should not be a deterrent to having surgery. In fact, the survival rate of the study's older participants was comparable to that of their peers who did not have surgery.[1]

At the same time, however, normal aging-related changes and diseases that occur more frequently in midlife, particularly heart problems, can sometimes make surgery more of a concern. Here are some tips from the National Institutes of Health for picking a surgeon:[2]

1. Check to see if the surgeon you select has been certified by a medical board. Surgeons who are board certified have had a number of years of training in dealing with certain diseases and have passed the examination for their specialty. Don't hesitate to call the doctor's office and ask for this information. Your state and local medical society and the hospital where the surgeon operates should also be able to verify his or her qualifications.

2. Another way of checking a surgeon's qualifications is to see if he or she is a Fellow of the American College of Surgeons. The letters F.A.C.S. after the surgeon's name

---

[1] "Too Old for Surgery?" *Arthritis Today*, January–February 1990

[2] Adapted from *Age Pages*, National Institute on Aging..

indicate that he or she has passed an evaluation of surgical training and skills as well as ethical fitness.

3. Choose an experienced surgeon who operates *at least* several times a week. The best surgeon to perform hysterectomies and related surgery is usually a *reproductive surgeon* who strives to operate in a way that cuts down on scars and adhesions.

4. Get a second opinion. For information on when and why you should consider getting a second opinion, write to the Health Care Financing Administration for the brochure "Thinking of Having Surgery?" The address is Surgery, HHS, Washington, DC 20201.

Ask questions. Before undergoing a surgical procedure, you will be asked to sign a statement giving consent for the operation. It is important that you discuss all your concerns about your condition and the operation with your surgeon before you sign this statement. If you are about to have a myomectomy, be sure to refer to Key 25 about how to fill out a consent form for this procedure, to prevent the removal of your reproductive organs.

The following checklist provides some basic questions for which you should have answers before you schedule your surgery:

• What does the doctor say your problem is?

• What is the operation the doctor plans to do?

• What will the results be if you don't have the operation?

• What will the results be if you have the operation?

• Are there other forms of treatment that could be tried before surgery?

• What are the risks of surgery?

• How long will the recovery period be and what is involved?

- How much will the operation cost? Will insurance cover all the costs, including special tests?

- How much experience has the surgeon had with this particular operation?

- What percentage of the operations were successful?

- Who will administer the anesthesia? Has the doctor or nurse anesthetist had experience treating older adults?

- How will the operation affect your lifestyle? Are there any activities you will not be able to do after surgery?

If You Are a Medicare Recipient

Medicare will cover the costs of a second opinion for elective surgery. And if the second opinion disagrees with the first, Medicare will also cover the cost of a third opinion. Medicare offers a second opinion hotline. The hotline operator will give you the name of a specialist in your area. The number is (800) 638-6833; in Maryland it is (800) 492-6603.

37

ESTROGEN AND HEART DISEASE

Most of us fear cancer as the major thief of life, whereas heart disease is the real culprit. The number one killer of women in the United States is heart disease, taking about 500,000 lives a year. However, heart disease rarely occurs in women before the menopause years. (The exception is for women who smoke and/or take birth control pills.) Researchers believe that estrogen is the protective factor. The hormone appears to raise HDL, the good cholesterol, which cleanses the blood of fatty deposits.

Because heart disease strikes men earlier in life than it affects women, it long has been considered a man's disease. However, some troubling new studies have shown that women are twice as likely as men to die within a year after having a heart attack and are at greater risk of having a second attack. Moreover, there is a tremendous gender gap in treatment. Part of the reason for this is that the instruments and procedures used for treatment, such as angioplasty, were designed for men, not women. Two recent studies reported that men are twice as likely as women to receive coronary angiography, which is an important diagnostic procedure, along with coronary bypass surgery.[1]

What is a woman to do? The good news is that women who can take estrogen supplements can significantly cut their risk of getting heart disease. The most recent finding is from an important project at Boston's Brigham and Women's Hospital, which is studying 48,470 nurses who are postmenopausal.

---

[1] Ron Winslow, "Women Face Treatment Gap in Heart Disease," *Wall Street Journal,* July 25, 1991, p. B1.

The research results strengthened the findings of a number of earlier studies and analyses. For example, a literature review that looked at 31 studies found that 25 of them showed that estrogen reduced coronary risk. And in 12 of these studies the reduction was statistically significant.[2]

Briefly, the results of the Boston study are:

- Women who take estrogen are almost half as likely as those who never took the supplement to have nonfatal heart attacks or to die from heart disease.

- The death rate from all causes is 19 percent lower among estrogen users.

However, the benefits wear off when estrogen is stopped. Therefore, to receive the protection of estrogen, you will have to take the hormone for the rest of your life.

The Progesterone Question

There is some speculation that taking progesterone with estrogen can cut down on estrogen's protection against heart disease. In fact, progesterone may raise the levels of LDL, the bad cholesterol, and lower the levels of HDL, the good cholesterol.

Unfortunately, none of the large studies have analyzed the effects of taking estrogen and progesterone together. However, the studies that have shown adverse effects of progesterone on HDL and LDL used a much higher dosage of progesterone than that now used in HRT.

Risk

You are at high risk for heart disease if you smoke, have high blood pressure, elevated cholesterol, and a family history of heart disease, or have had your ovaries removed.

---

[2]M. J. Stampfer and G. A. Colditz, "Estrogen Replacement Therapy and Coronary Heart Disease: A Quantitative Assessment of the Epidemiologic Evidence," *Preventive Medicine,* vol. 20, issue 1, January 1991, pp. 47–63.

Preventing Heart Disease

Estrogen is not the only deterrent to heart disease to receive wide attention. A preliminary study conducted at Brigham and Women's Hospital and Harvard Medical School in Boston suggest that women receive the same benefit from taking aspirin to prevent heart disease as men do. Their report says that women over age 50 who took from one to six aspirin a week were 32 percent less likely to have a heart attack than women who took no aspirin. Doctors recommend taking one baby aspirin a day. (Taking more will not increase the benefit but can cause stomach problems.) Other important preventive measures for heart disease include the following:

Don't smoke.

Check your blood pressure regularly. If your blood pressure is high, take measures to get it down.

Eat a balanced diet, low in fat. (See Key 40.)

Keep your weight down.

Exercise regularly. (See Key 39.)

Try techniques to relax. (See Key 42.)

Take any preventive medicines prescribed by your physician.

38

WHAT TO EXPECT DURING YOUR YEARLY GYNECOLOGICAL EXAMINATION

Because problems in the reproductive system are more likely to occur once you reach midlife, it is important to have a yearly gynecological examination. The examination can be performed by a gynecologist, internist, family practitioner, or qualified nurse practitioner. However, generalists such as internists or family practitioners should refer you to specialists for problems that they are not familiar handling.

A key factor in the success of your medical care is whether you relate well to your health care provider. It is important to feel that you can be open about even the most embarrassing of symptoms, including signs of incontinence, vaginal discharges, and sagging tissue.

Your yearly gynecological exam should be accompanied by monthly breast self-examinations (see Key 30). Moreover, you should make sure that your doctor is highly experienced in performing breast exams. Even the most experienced physician can miss cancerous growths, particularly in breasts that tend to be naturally lumpy.

It is always a good rule of thumb to write down any questions you may have, before arriving at the doctor's office. If you feel that your doctor is not giving you enough time, find another health care provider. The point of your yearly examination is to *discuss* and *investigate* any problems you may be having. If you are prevented from doing this, you are not getting thorough care.

Your annual exam should include the doctor's standard procedures, such as a blood pressure check and an exam with a stethoscope. In addition, the following must be included: breast and pelvic exams, a Pap test, and a rectal exam. Breast and Pap tests are covered in other sections of this book. The following discussion will provide details on the pelvic and rectal exams.

The Pelvic Exam

Your doctor will examine your outer genital area to check for infection and other problems. Then, a speculum will be inserted to spread apart your vaginal walls and check your vaginal lining for signs of growths or other problems. The doctor will take a Pap smear while the speculum is in place.

The doctor will then perform an internal examination of your ovaries, uterus, and fallopian tubes. To accomplish this, the physician will insert two fingers in your vagina, while pressing the other hand against the outside of your lower abdomen.

The Rectal Exam

Your doctor will use a similar technique to perform a rectal examination. Inserting the index finger in the vagina and middle finger in the rectum, the physician will check your rectum.

Medical Providers You May Encounter

Usually the best way to locate a physician with whom you can relate well is by personal referrals. Ask your doctors, your friends, and check with local referral services. The following provides details on the types of doctors you may see for your annual exam and routine gynecological care:

- *Doctors of medicine (M.D.s)* treat diseases and injuries, provide preventive care, do routine checkups, prescribe drugs, and perform some surgery. M.D.s complete medical school plus three to seven years of graduate medical education. They must be licensed in the state in which they practice.

- *Internists* are M.D.s who specialize in the diagnosis and medical treatment of disease in adults. Internists do not perform surgery or deliver babies.

- *Family practitioners* are M.D.s who specialize in providing comprehensive health care for all members of a family, regardless of age or sex, on a continuing basis.

- *Doctors of osteopathic medicine (D.O.s)* provide general health care to individuals and families. The training they receive is similar to that of an M.D. In addition to drugs, surgery, and other treatments, a D.O. may manipulate muscles and bones to treat specific problems.

- *Gynecologists* are M.D.s who specialize in the female reproductive system.

In addition, you may see these health professionals:

- *Physician assistants (P.A.s)* do physical examinations, take medical histories, carry out diagnostic tests, and develop treatment plans for patients. Their education includes two to four years of college followed by a two-year period of special training. P.A.s must always be under the supervision of a doctor, but, depending on state laws, the supervision can be by telephone rather than in person. In some states, P.A.s can prescribe certain drugs.

- *Nurse practitioners (R.N.s, N.P.s)* are registered nurses with training beyond basic nursing education. Nurse practitioners perform physical examinations and diagnostic tests, counsel patients, and develop treatment programs. Regulations regarding their duties vary from state to state. Nurse practitioners may work independently, such as in rural clinics, or may be staff members at hospitals and other health facilities.

- *Registered nurses (R.N.s)* may have two, three, or four years of education in a nursing school. In addition to performing bedside nursing duties, such as giving medicine, administering treatments, and educating patients, R.N.s also work in doctors' offices, clinics, and community health agencies.

In addition, you may see these medical specialists to treat specific problems:

- *Endocrinologists* treat disorders of the glands of internal secretion, such as hormone problems.

- *Oncologists* treat tumors and cancer.

- *Orthopedists* treat problems relating to osteoporosis and bones, muscles, ligaments, and tendons.

- *Urologists* treat the urinary system.

To check the credentials of a doctor in your area, the American Board of Medical Specialties has a hotline for consumers that answers questions about a doctor's area of specialty and whether he or she is board certified. The number is 1-800-776-CERT. In addition, you can check out the credentials of doctors through the *Directory of Medical Specialists* in your local library.

39

EXERCISE

Hippocrates, living five centuries before Christ, was one of the first to understand the value of exercise to hinder the march of time. He said

All parts of the body which have a function, if used in moderation and exercised in labors to which each is accustomed, become thereby well-developed and age slowly; but if unused and left idle, they become liable to disease, defective in growth, and age quickly.

If your response to exercise is "I'm too old to start now," think twice. Exercise—started at any age, even after a long period of inactivity—has benefits. Maximum oxygen consumption (VO2 max) is an example. The greater a person's VO2 the greater his or her endurance. Studies have shown that, even if an older person has been inactive previously, an aerobic exercise program results in an average increase in VO2 max of 10 to 30 percent.

Aerobic exercise. This Key covers the benefits of aerobic exercise in general and, specifically, the benefits of walking. Aerobic exercise improves overall fitness and includes walking, stationary bicycling, swimming, and low-impact aerobics classes. In order for exercise to be aerobic, your pulse must be within the target heart rate for your age. The target zone is 60 to 75 percent of your maximum workout rate during vigorous exercise. The following will help you figure out your maximum rate:

To take your pulse, press your index (second) finger and third finger of one hand firmly against the wrist just below the thumb side of the other hand. Count the beats for fifteen seconds, then multiply by four. To figure your maximum

rate, subtract your age from the number 220. When exercising, your heart should not beat more times per minute than this number and it should be in the range of 60 to 75 percent of the maximum workout rate. For example, if you are age 50 your maximum workout rate is 170 beats per minute and the range that you should be in is 102 to 143 beats per minute. Your target zone should never go below 100 beats per minute.

For aerobic fitness your pulse should reach this rate for 20 to 30 minutes at least three times a week. However, you should work up to this amount in five-minute increments. The exercise program should include a warm-up, conditioning exercise, and a cool-down.

Most experts recommend that every aerobic session have a warm-up and cool-down period of three to five minutes before and after aerobic exercise of any kind. The intensity of these periods should be halfway between the previous activity and the aerobic activity. Slow walking, light calisthenics, and stretching are warm-up activities.

Walking. Walking is highly recommended to prevent osteoporosis, is one of the most readily available exercises for people of all ages, and has the distinct advantage of being free. For most older people, walking will result in a target heart zone that is intense enough to be aerobic if performed for a long enough time. For many older people, walking for half an hour to an hour three times a week is aerobic. Follow these tips from the Public Health Service to get started on a regular regimen:

- Wear comfortable shoes with good arch supports. They should be made of materials that breathe, like leather or nylon.
- Take long strides at a steady pace. Hold your head erect, back straight, and stomach flat. Point your toes straight ahead and let your arms swing loosely at your sides.

- Start a regular routine by walking every other day for about 15 minutes. Warm up by walking slowly for about five minutes, then faster for five minutes. Then cool down by walking slowly for the last five.
- Listen to your body. Brisk walking should make your heart beat faster and your breathing deeper. But stop if you find yourself panting, feeling nauseous, or unable to get your breathing back to normal within ten minutes.
- Gradually increase your distance and the length of your stride. In five weeks, you should be walking about a mile and ready to increase the frequency of your walking to five times a week. Continue five minutes of slow walking at the beginning and the end, but extend your brisk walking period.
- Add a time and distance goal to your walking sessions. After seven weeks, try walking a mile in 20 minutes. Next, increase your distance and stick to the 20-minute goal. A good goal to work up to (over about 15 weeks) is walking three miles in 45 minutes.
- Remember good walking form. Land on the heel of your foot and move forward to spring off the ball. You'll tire or become sore more quickly if you walk only on the balls of your feet or are flat-footed.

40

EATING RIGHT

Calcium and Osteoporosis

Including calcium in your daily diet is an important way to guard against osteoporosis. Foods rich in calcium include milk, yogurt, cheese and other dairy products, dark green leafy vegetables, canned salmon, and other foods. As mentioned in Key 17 you should have 1,200 to 1,500 milligrams of calcium a day to avoid osteoporosis. Table 1 lists some good sources of calcium.

The "sun" vitamin, vitamin D, is also one of the keys to preventing osteoporosis. It can be found in sunshine and milk. However, too much vitamin D can cause as many problems as too little. If you do not eat or drink many dairy products or get much sun, ask your doctor's advice on whether you should take a vitamin D supplement.

The Effect of Medicines on Diet

If you are taking any medication, it is important to check with your doctor to see how it may affect your nutrition. For example, many diuretics rob the body of potassium, and corticosteroids often cause weight gain and redistribution. Aspirin causes excretion of vitamin C in urine. On the other side of the coin, some medications contain too much of certain nutrients such as sodium, which can lead to hypertension, heart disease, and other conditions. Antacids, as well as steroids, for example, are high in sodium.

Basics of Nutrition

As people age, the body's basic need for nutrients, such as proteins, carbohydrates, vitamins, and minerals, is not different than when we were young. However, the body's need for calories *decreases* because of physical changes and decreasing activity. The result is that many people put on weight.

Table 1.

Some Calcium-Rich Foods			
	Measure	**Calories**	**Calcium (mg)**
Dairy			
Cheese			
Blue	1 ounce	100	**150**
Cheddar, cut pieces	1 ounce	115	**204**
Feta	1 ounce	75	**140**
Mozzarella made with whole milk	1 ounce	80	**147**
Mozzarella, made with part skim milk	1 ounce	80	**207**
Muenster	1 ounce	105	**203**
Parmesan	1 tbsp	25	**69**
Pasteurized process American	1 ounce	105	**174**
Swiss	1 ounce	95	**219**
Provolone	1 ounce	100	**214**
Swiss	1 ounce	105	**272**
Cottage Cheese			
Lowfat (2%)	1 cup	205	**155**
Creamed (4% fat) Large curd	1 cup	235	**135**
Small curd	1 cup	215	**126**
Milk			
Skim	1 cup	85	**302**
1% fat	1 cup	100	**300**
2% fat	1 cup	120	**297**
Whole (3.3% fat)	1 cup	150	**291**
Buttermilk	1 cup	100	**285**
Dry, nonfat, instant	¼ cup	61	**209**

	Measure	**Calories**	**Calcium (mg)**
Yogurt			
Plain, lowfat, with added milk solids	8 ounces	145	**415**
Fruit flavored, lowfat, with added milk solids	8 ounces	230*	**345***
Plain, whole milk	8 ounces	140	**274**
Dairy Desserts			
Custard, baked	1 cup	305	**297**
Ice cream, vanilla Regular (11% fat)			
Hardened	1 cup	270	**176**
Soft serve	1 cup	375	**236**
Ice milk, vanilla			
Hardened, 4% fat	1 cup	185	**176**
Soft serve, 3% fat	1 cup	225	**274**
Seafood			
Oysters, raw, meat only (13–19 medium)	1 cup	160	**226**
Salmon, pink, canned, *including the bones*	3 ounces	120	**167****
Sardines, Atlantic, canned in oil, drained, *including the bones*	3 ounces	175	**371****
Shrimp, canned, drained, solids	3 ounces	100	**98**

* These values may vary.
** If the bones are discarded, the amount of calcium is greatly reduced.

	Measure	Calories	Calcium (mg)
Vegetables			
Bok choy, raw, chopped	1 cup	9	**74**
Broccoli, raw	1 spear	40	**72**
Broccoli, cooked, drained, from raw, ½" pieces	1 cup	45	**177**
Broccoli, cooked, drained, from frozen, chopped	1 cup	50	**94**
Collards, cooked, drained, from frozen	1 cup	60	**357**
Dandelion greens, cooked, drained	1 cup	35	**147**
Kale, cooked, drained, from frozen	1 cup	40	**179**
Mustard greens, without stems and midribs, cooked, drained	1 cup	20	**104**
Turnip greens, chopped, cooked, drained, from frozen	1 cup	50	**249**
Dried Beans			
Cooked, drained			
Great Northern	1 cup	210	**90**
Navy	1 cup	225	**95**
Pinto	1 cup	265	**86**
Chickpeas (garbanzos), cooked, drained	1 cup	270	**80**
Red kidney, canned	1 cup	230	**74**

	Measure	Calories	Calcium (mg)
Refried beans, canned	1 cup	295	**141**
Soy beans, cooked, drained	1 cup	235	**131**
Miscellaneous			
Molasses, cane, blackstrap	2 tbsp	85	**274**
Tofu, 2 ½" x 2 ¾" x 1" (about 4 ounces	1 piece	85*	**108***

* Both of these values may vary, especially the calcium content, depending on how the tofu is made. Tofu processed with calcium salts can have as much as 300 mg calcium per 4 ounces. The label, your grocer, or the manufacturer can provide more specific information.

Source: U.S. Department of Health and Human Services, Public Health Service, National Institutes on Health

The National Institute on Aging (NIA), part of the National Institutes on Health, points out that as people get older they should limit their intake of fatty foods, sweets, salty snack foods, high-calorie drinks, and alcohol. These foods are high in calories, but *not* nutrients.

NIA points out that a nutritious diet provides minerals, vitamins, and calories from proteins, carbohydrates, and some fats. Such a diet must include a variety of foods from all the major food groups: fruits and vegetables; whole grain and enriched breads, cereals, and grain products such as rice and pasta; fish, poultry, meats, eggs, and dry beans and peas; and milk, cheese, and other dairy products.

Limiting the amount of fat in the diet may help prevent weight gain. Limiting fat may also help protect against heart disease and breast cancer. NIA also recommends reducing salt intake.

The following is a list of the major nutrients that you should include in your diet:

Protein. This is the basic material in all body cells. It also enables growth and repair of body cells and helps the body resist disease.

During digestion, food proteins are broken down into simple nutrients called amino acids, which are the building blocks of life. The body then reassembles these proteins into the types of proteins it needs.

Many foods contain protein. The proteins in meats, fish, dairy products, and eggs contain the essential amino acids in proper amounts for adults. These are complete proteins. The easiest way to get complete amino acids is to eat some of these foods every day. Plant foods such as dry peas and beans, grains, nuts, and seeds contain "incomplete" proteins, because not all the essential amino acids are present. However, when one of these foods is combined with an animal protein (milk and cereal, for example) or when certain plant proteins are combined (such as rice with beans), they form complete proteins. Foods high in protein also provide essential vitamins and minerals.

Carbohydrates. There are two types of carbohydrates. *Complex* carbohydrates are starches present in grains, cereals, legumes, potatoes, and other vegetables, and sugars present in fruits and milk. These foods are good sources of vitamins, minerals, fiber, and calories. *Simple* sugars are found in desserts, candy, honey, syrup, and other sugary foods. These are the foods that we love to eat but have to limit, since they provide few nutrients.

Breads and cereals are more nutritious if made from whole grains. Such products include whole wheat and rye breads and crackers, whole wheat cereals, bran, oatmeal, barley, brown rice, and cornmeal.

Fats. Fats are concentrated sources of calories. Some fat is needed in the diet because it provides essential amino acids and gives flavor to food. However, the typical American diet is too high in fat and cholesterol. Low-fat foods include fish, poultry, lean meats, dry beans and peas, skim milk, yogurt, buttermilk, fruits, vegetables, and grains. Eggs and organ meats should be limited, as well as butter, cream, mayonnaise, margarine, oils, lard, certain prepared foods (for example, fast-food hamburgers), and snack food such as potato chips.

Vitamins and minerals. These are needed by the body in relatively small amounts. The fat-soluble vitamins A, D, E, and K are absorbed along with fat from various foods and are stored in the body. The water-soluble vitamins, the B's and C, generally are not stored. Minerals such as calcium, phosphorus, iron, iodine, magnesium, and zinc are also required for building body tissues and regulating their functions.

Vitamins and minerals are abundant in fruits, vegetables, meats, dairy products, and whole grain or enriched breads and cereals.

Fiber. Another important part of the diet is fiber, which is present in foods that grow. The role of fiber is not known for sure, but it can help prevent constipation, intestinal disorders, and cancer of the colon.

The best way to include fiber in the diet is to eat whole grain breads and cereals and plenty of vegetables and fruits. Adding a few tablespoons of unprocessed bran, which is high in fiber, to cereal and other foods is acceptable. However, excessive intake of bran can decrease the body's absorption of minerals such as iron and calcium. Table 2 lists some good sources of fiber.

Table 2.

Sources of Fiber		
Food	Serving Size	Grams of Fiber
Cereals		
All or 100% Bran	⅓–½ cup (1 oz)	8.4–8.5
Bran Buds	⅓ cup (1 oz)	7.9
Bran Chex	⅔ cup (1 oz)	4.6
Corn Bran	⅔ cup (1 oz)	5.4
40% Bran-type	¾ cup (1 oz)	4.0
Extra Fiber Bran Cereal	½ cup (1 oz)	12–13
HoneyBran	⅞ cup (1 oz)	3.1
Most	⅔ cup (1 oz)	3.5
Raisin Bran-type	¾ cup (1 oz)	4.0
Shredded Wheat	⅔ cup (1 oz)	2.6
Wheat 'n' Raisin Chex	¾ cup (1⅓ oz)	2.5
Wheat germ	¼ cup (2 oz)	3.4
Bread, Pasta, Grains		
Bran muffins	1 regular muffin	2.5
Cracked wheat bread	1 slice	1.0
Pumpernickel bread	1 slice	1.0
Whole wheat bread	1 slice	1.4
Crisp bread, rye	2 crackers	2.0
Crisp bread, wheat	2 crackers	1.8
Rice, brown	½ cup (cooked)	1.0
Spaghetti, whole wheat	1 cup (cooked)	3.9
Popcorn	1 cup	2.5

Food	Serving Size	Grams of Fiber
Fruits		
Apple (w/skin)	1 medium	3.5
Apple (w/o skin)	1 medium	2.7
Banana	1 medium	2.4
Orange	1	2.6
Pear (w/skin)	½ large	3.1
Pear (w/o skin)	½ large	2.5
Prunes	3	3.0
Raisins	¼ cup	3.1
Raspberries	½ cup	3.1
Strawberries	1 cup	3.0
Vegetables, cooked		
Broccoli	½ cup	2.2
Brussels sprouts	½ cup	2.3
Carrots	½ cup	2.3
Corn, canned	½ cup	2.9
Parsnip	½ cup	2.7
Peas	½ cup	3.6
Potato (w/skin)	1 medium	2.5
Spinach	½ cup	2.1
Sweet potato	½ medium	1.7
Zucchini	½ cup	1.8
Beans, Legumes		
Baked beans, tomato sauce	½ cup	8.8
Kidney beans, cooked	½ cup	7.3
Lima beans, cooked/canned	½ cup	4.5
Navy beans, cooked	½ cup	6.0
Lentils	½ cup	3.7

Source: The American Institute for Cancer Research, © 1989.

41

SEXUALITY AND BIRTH CONTROL

This Key covers three important aspects of sex in midlife: women and sexual *desire*, sex-related *changes* that can occur in males, and *birth control*.

Women and Sexual Desire

Is there sex after midlife? Yes! Many research studies have found that midlife and older people enjoy active sex lives. One study of 4,000 people conducted by the Consumers Union Foundation found that two-thirds of women over 70 enjoyed active sex lives. Experts say that women and men who enjoy regular sexual activity throughout their adult lives are most apt to continue enjoying regular sexual activity during their older years.

However, sexual changes do occur. As mentioned in Key 10, sex after menopause can become uncomfortable because of changes in the vagina. Another important factor is sex drive, which decreases for some women. However, other women report that they are more interested in sex after menopause.

If your desire for sex is not what it used to be, it may be the result of low levels of testosterone. Produced by the ovaries, this hormone increases the libido. You may want to ask your doctor about having your androgen level checked. If it is low, your physician can prescribe very low doses of testosterone. This is also an important option for women who have had their ovaries removed. (Many women worry that because testosterone is known as a male hormone, it will cause masculinizing characteristics. However, when taken in low doses, this is not the case.)

Sex-Related Changes in Males

Sexual changes also occur for men. Lower testosterone levels may lower their desire for sex. They may take longer to attain an erection than when they were younger, and the erection may not be as firm or as large. There can be a shorter sensation that an ejaculation is about to occur. The loss of erection following orgasm may be more rapid, followed by a longer waiting period before an erection is possible again.

Birth Control

A general rule of thumb is that birth control should be used at least up to the time your periods end. Many doctors recommend continuing birth control for a year after the last period. However, women over 35 should not be taking birth control pills, particularly if they smoke. The rhythm method of birth control may be difficult to carry out during this time, because ovulation is unpredictable.

42

REST AND RELAXATION

Along with nutrition and exercise, rest and relaxation are important to adjusting to the changes that take place during menopause. This Key covers some basic relaxation techniques to enable you to regain serenity during times of stress.

Deep Breathing. This is a technique for averting shallow, ineffective breathing by learning to breathe deeply and slowly. It is a part of many other relaxation techniques.

Autogenic relaxing. In this approach you talk yourself into relaxing. For example, you first get comfortable and then progressively tell different parts of your body to relax: "My toes are now relaxed. The balls of my feet are now relaxed...."

Biofeedback. This technique can teach you how to relax by giving you "feedback" from specific body responses that tell when you are relaxed versus when you are tense. During biofeedback you are hooked up to electric equipment that monitors these physical reactions and gives you information on them. (You will not be shocked by the electricity.) This technique is very useful for people who have a hard time knowing when their body is relaxed.

Focusing. Based on research at the University of Chicago, this technique involves learning to identify the way personal problems manifest themselves in the body. It is becoming so popular some nursing schools are teaching it. In focusing you make contact with an internal bodily awareness through six specific movements. The technique is taught in a book called, appropriately, *Focusing* by Eugene T. Gendlin, published by Everest House or Bantam Books.

Imagery/creative visualization. This technique uses mental imagery to improve health and attitudes and block pain perception. The individual visualizes a favorite place that is associated with peaceful feelings or makes one up, such as floating on a cloud. The classic book showing how to use imagery is *Creative Visualization* by Shakti Gawain, published by New Age Bantam books.

Meditation. This technique involves concentrating on one sound or thought in order to reach a relaxed, peaceful state. When the technique is used properly, breathing will slow down and other physical signs of relaxation will be present. Meditation tapes are available in most book stores.

Prayer. For many, prayer is a way of relaxing and reaching a peaceful state of mind.

Progressive muscle relaxation. This technique teaches the difference between tight and relaxed muscles by alternately tensing and relaxing muscles. However, you should not attempt it if you have arthritic joints, as tightening could be bad for them.

QUESTIONS THAT MEN ASK

My husband and I were at our mountain retreat recently with friends of ours, when the topic of this book came up. Interestingly, it was the husband who was most interested in the subject from the standpoint of what his wife would one day be facing and what impact her menopause would have on their relationship. "What a loving attitude!" I thought. At the same time I realized anew how much the changes that come with menopause affect both partners in an ongoing relationship.

The following questions and answers are based on that discussion. I suggest showing this to the man in your life, particularly if he is a steady sex partner and you are normally reluctant to discuss these issues.

Q. Will my wife's (or significant other's) libido be affected?

A. Speaking strictly in terms of desire and enjoyment, the answer to this question is, "It depends on your wife." Many women report a welcome, relaxed feeling about sex and sexuality after menopause because they no longer have to fear pregnancy. The bad news, however, is that others report a waning libido during and after menopause; in other words, they notice a marked lack of interest in sexual intercourse. Additionally, as we will discuss in a minute, physical change in the genitourinary organs can also make the sexual act uncomfortable, and therefore, unpleasant. But, first let's talk about the decrease in libido.

A decreased libido can be the result of a number of problems, including attitude. Some women, for example, expect to lose interest in sex at midlife, and therefore, do. Others, however, don't produce enough of the hormone testosterone, which is responsible for one's sex drive. This could be a problem for the woman in your life if she has had her ovaries removed. (All women normally produce testosterone in their ovaries and adrenal glands.)

The good news for women who do not produce enough testosterone is that their doctors can prescribe low levels of the hormone to boost their desire for sex. Some estrogen replacement preparations even add low levels of testosterone to the estrogen dosage.

Finally, low or oscillating levels of estrogen can also cause sexual desire to skid. This is usually cleared up by taking hormone replacement therapy.

Q. Will our sex life be affected?

A. If your wife is not on hormone replacement therapy, your sex life will probably be affected in a number of ways. We just discussed libido. Another factor that can alter the quality and frequency of sexual intercourse is that marked changes occur in the vagina and genitals after menopause. These changes happen to all women who do not take estrogen, and they can cause pain or discomfort during sexual intercourse. Specifically, the external genitals and vagina (vulva) thin out and shrink when estrogen levels decrease. Sometimes the vagina actually shortens and becomes narrower. Pubic hair also thins. Vaginal secretions become less acidic and dryness, burning, itching, and vaginitis can result. Blood flow to the genitals decreases and some women actually have a narrowing of the entrance to the vagina so that intercourse is impossible. Lubrication also is slower. And the vagina becomes far more susceptible to infection.

These changes progress and, without estrogen, a thinning vagina may become so irritated by sex that it becomes undesirable. Happily, even if your partner has not taken estrogen for years and her vagina has seriously atrophied, estrogen will restore it to a functioning level.

And there is more good news. Many other things can be done to keep the genital area young and healthy. Lubricants, for example, can help to make sex less painful and more satisfying when the vagina is dry. Some doctors prescribe estrogen or testosterone cream for vaginal dryness. (However, both are medications and should not be applied for lovemaking only.)

The bottom line is that if you notice anything different about your partner, such as a vagina that is tighter or drier, talk to her about it. It is entirely possible that she does not notice it herself and she should discus it with her gynecologist.

Q. In regard to sex is there something we should or should not do?

A. You're going to like the answer to this question. One of the best things that you can do to keep your sex life going is— keep your sex life going. Sex literally aids the muscle tone of the vagina and keeps it elastic, flexible, and lubricated. And, according to Dr. Lila E. Nachtigall, any method of achieving orgasm is useful, as is using mechanical aids to tone and shape the vaginal walls if intercourse is not possible.[1]

It is important to understand that you may notice a change in your partner's responsiveness or sexuality and easily misinterpret it. For example, if your partner is not getting as much pleasure from your sex life as she used to, it may be because her hormone levels are dipping. It may have nothing to do with you. Again, the two of you should talk this over.

Q. What help can men give their partners?

A. This is an easy question with a short answer. Be supportive. Menopause is often associated with a myriad of symptoms that may make your partner uncomfortable. The best thing that you can do is make her feel loved, attractive, and appreciated.

---

[1] Lila E. Nachtigall, *Estrogen*, HarperPerennial, 1991, p 91.

Q. Will my partner's health be affected?

A. Yes, estrogen provides women with a number of protections that are lost when hormone levels decrease during and after menopause. For example, women who do not take estrogen are twice as likely as those who do to have nonfatal heart attacks or to die from heart disease. Second, menopausal women are highly susceptible to developing osteoporosis, a condition in which bone mass decreases, causing them to fracture easily.

Happily, researchers agree that both heart disease and osteoporosis are highly preventable through taking estrogen, exercising regularly, and taking in adequate calcium. And, for those women who cannot take estrogen, there are important things they *can* do.

Many men worry about their partners taking estrogen because of the fear of cancer. However, there is no evidence of a relationship between menopausal estrogen therapy and breast cancer.[2] Many doctors believe that estrogen helps protect against cancer of the ovary, a more serious disease than uterine cancer.[3] And with the addition of progesterone the risk of developing uterine cancer has been greatly reduced. In fact, women who take estrogen have lower death rates from all causes than those who do not.

Q. What are the major symptoms that my partner and I should watch out for?

A. Some lucky women never have real problems with menopause. However, most women will experience at least three or four of the major signs of menopause listed below. (Details of these symptoms are described in Keys 9 through 17.)

---

[2]Council on Scientific Affairs, "Estrogen Replacement in the Menopause," *Journal of the American Medical Association,* Jan. 21, 1983, Vol. 249, No. 3.

[3]Niels Laursen and Steven Whitney, *A Woman's Body: The New Guide to Gynecology,* Perigree, 1987, p 431.

- hot flashes or flushes
- changes in menstruation
- vaginal changes
- stress incontinence
- weight gain
- skin and hair changes
- premenstrual syndrome (PMS)
- sleep changes
- mood swings
- osteoporosis

I'd like to talk a little bit about sleep changes, because after hot flashes, the inability to sleep at night (insomnia) is the second most frequent menopause-related complaint.[4] And if your mate is experiencing menopause-related insomnia and is up and down during the night, pacing the halls in an attempt to wear herself out, you may both have blood-shot eyes in the morning. Fortunately, there are many things that can be done to aid your partner's insomnia, including, once again, estrogen replacement therapy. (For other suggestions, see Key 15 of this book.) And the condition is usually relatively short term, lasting only through the peak years of the condition.

Q. How does menopause affect reproduction? Can the woman in my life still get pregnant?

A. A general rule of thumb is that birth control should be used at least up to the time your partner's periods end. And many doctors recommend continuing birth control for a year after the last period.

---

[4]Lila E. Nachtigall and Joan Rattner Heilman, *Estrogen,* HarperPerennial, 1991, 65.

GLOSSARY

Amenorrhea absence of menstruation.

Anovulatory without eggs.

Areola the pigmented ring around the nipple of the breast.

Biopsy a medical procedure in which a sample of tissue is removed for examination under a microscope.

Cervix the end of the uterus that extends into the vagina.

D and C (dilatation and curettage) a procedure in which the opening of the cervix is stretched and an instrument is inserted to scrape away the uterine lining.

Dyspareunia painful sexual intercourse.

Dysplasia impaired growth processes.

Endometrium the mucous membrane lining of the uterus.

Estrogen a female hormone that is produced in the ovaries.

Fibroid tumor swelling or growth, usually not cancerous.

Genitourinary the sex organs and the urinary system.

Hormone Replacement Therapy (HRT) a treatment in which estrogen and often progesterone are taken.

Hormones substances that are produced by the body to control functions.

Hypothalamus a portion of the brain that sends messages to the pituitary gland to stimulate the ovary.

In situ describes cancer in early stages, in one area.

Laparoscopy examining the abdominal cavity through the use of a lighted instrument.

Lymph nodes small, bean-shaped organs located along the lymphatic system. Also called lymph glands.

Malignant cancerous (tumors).

Mammography X-ray examination of the breast.

Melanoma a cancer derived from cells containing pigment.

Menopause the term used to describe that specific point in time when you had your last period.

Myomectomy the surgical removal of fibroid tumors from the uterus.

Osteoporosis a condition in which the bones become weak.

Ovaries two small organs located on either side of the uterus. They produce eggs and the female sex hormones, estrogen and progesterone.

Pathologist a doctor who identifies diseases by studying cells and tissues under a microscope.

Pessary a plastic or rubber appliance that fits in the vagina and holds the uterus, bladder, and other organs in place.

pH denotes alkalinity or acidity.

Polyps growths of mucous membranes.

Progesterone a female hormone that is produced in the ovaries and prepares the lining of the uterus to nourish a fertilized egg.

Progestin a synthetic form of progesterone.

Prolapse the falling out of position of an organ.

Pruritus the medical term for itching skin in the vulva or genital areas.

Remodeling a process where bone is broken down and remade.

Senile vaginitis itching in the genital area, plus a discharge.

Sonography a diagnostic method using sound waves to create an image with a computer.

Speculum an instrument inserted in a body opening to look inside

Stress incontinence the loss of urine with activities that put pressure on the bladder.

Urge incontinence the loss of urine that occurs whenever there is a strong desire to urinate.

Uterus a pear-shaped organ about the size of a lemon. It carries the fetus during pregnancy.

Vagina the canal lying between the rectum and bladder. It is the area of the body where sexual intercourse occurs, and it stretches easily during sex or childbirth.

RESOURCES

Organizations
American Board of Medical Specialties
One Rotary Center, Suite 805
Evanston, IL 60201
(800) 776-CERT

American Board of Obstetrics and Gynecology
4225 Roosevelt Way NW, Suite 305
Seattle, WA 98105
(206) 547-4884

American Cancer Society
1599 Clifton Rd. NE
Atlanta, GA 30329
(404) 320-3333

American College of Obstetricians and Gynecologists
409 12th St. SW
Washington, DC
(202) 638-5577

Boston Women's Health Collective
240 A Elm St.
Somerville, MA 02114
(617) 625-0271

Calcium Information Center
Cornell University Medical Center
(800) 321-2681

Cancer Information Service
(800) 4-CANCER

Hysterectomy Educational Resources and Services
HERS Foundation
422 Bryn Mawr Ave.
Bala Cynwyd, PA 19004
(215) 667-7757

National Osteoporosis Foundation
2100 M St. NW, Suite 602
Washington, DC 20037
(202) 223-2226

National Women's Health Network
1325 G St. NW
Washington DC 20005
(202) 347-1140

National Women's Health Resource Center
2440 M St. NW
Washington DC
(202) 293-6045

OWL (Older Women's League)
666 11th St. NW, Suite 700
Washington DC 20001
(202) 783-6686

Planned Parenthood Federation of America
810 Seventh Ave.
New York, NY 10019
(212) 541-7800

Newsletters
Menopause News, 2074 Union Street, Suite 10, San Francisco, CA 94123.

Hot Flash Newsletter, National Action Forum for Midlife and Older Women, PO Box 816, Stony Brook, NY 11790-0609.

INDEX

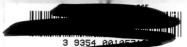

3 9354 001